Urological Complications of Pelvic Surgery and Radiotherapy

Urological Complications of Pelvic Surgery and Radiotherapy

Edited by

Michael A. S. Jewett

Professor and Chairman,
Division of Urology,
University of Toronto,
The Toronto Hospital,
200 Elizabeth Street,
Toronto, Canada

I S I S
MEDICAL
MEDIA
—
Oxford

© 1995 by Isis Medical Media Ltd
Saxon Beck, 58 St Aldates
Oxford OX1 1ST, UK

First published 1995

British Library Cataloguing in Publication Data. A catalogue record for this title is available from the British Library

ISBN 1 899066 14 4

Jewett (Michael A.S.)
Urological Complications of Pelvic Surgery and Radiotherapy/
Michael A S Jewett

Always refer to the manufacturer's Prescribing Information before prescribing drugs cited in this book.

Set by
Marksbury Typesetting Ltd, Midsomer Norton, Bath, UK

Printed by
Biddles Ltd, Guildford & Kings Lynn, UK

Distributed by
Times Mirror International Publishers, Customer Service Centre, Unit 1, 3 Sheldon Way, Larkfield, Aylesford, Kent ME20 6SF, UK

Contents

List of Contributors

Klaus Bandhauer Prof. MD
Chief of Department of Urology, Kantonsspital St Gallen, Switzerland

Michele Battaglia MD
Senior Urologist, Chair of Urology 'R', University of Bari, Policlinico, 70 124 Bari, Italy

Véronique Beckendorf MD
Senior Consultant, Radiotherapy Department, Centre Alexis Vautrin, Avenue de Bourgogne, 54511 Vandoeuvre les Nancy, Cedex, France

Nabil K. Bissada MD
Professor and Chief of Urologic Oncology, Department of Urology, Medical University of South Carolina, 171 Ashley Avenue, Charleston, SC, 29425, USA

Juan L. Casanova-Ramon MD
Consultant, Department of Urology, Instituto Valenciano de Oncología, C/- Prof. Beltran Baguena, 19, 46009 Valencia, Spain

Christopher R. Chapple BSc MD FRCS(Urol)
Consultant Urological Surgeon, Department of Urology, The Royal Hallamshire Hospital, Glossop Road, Sheffield, S10 2JF, UK

Luigi Cormio MD
Urologist, Chair of Urology 'R', University of Bari, Policlinico, 70 124 Bari, Italy

Raimundo Dumont-Martinez MD PhD
Consultant, Department of Urology, Instituto Valenciano de Oncología, C/- Prof. Beltran Baguena, 19, 46009 Valencia, Spain

Oliver W. Hakenberg MD
Senior Registrar, Department of Surgery, Flinders Medical Centre, Bedford Park, South Australia, 5041, Australia

Inmaculada Iborra-Juan MD PhD
Consultant, Department of Urology, Instituto Valenciano de Oncología, C/- Prof. Beltran Baguena, 19, 46009 Valencia, Spain

Morrie S. Liquornik MFCM FRCS(C)
Fellow, Department of Surgery, Division of Urology, The Toronto Hospital, Western Division, Toronto, Canada

José López-Torrecilla   MD Radiotherapy
Assistant, Department of Radiotherapy, Instituto Valenciano de Oncología, C/- Prof.
Beltran Baguena, 19, 46009 Valencia, Spain

Ulrich Maier   MD
Associate Professor of Urology, Department of Urology, University of Vienna,
Währinger Gürtel 18-20, A-1090, Vienna, Austria

Stephan Madersbacher   MD
Department of Urology, University of Vienna, Währinger Gürtel 18-20, A-1090
Vienna, Austria

Michael Marberger   MD
Professor and Chairman, Department of Urology, University of Vienna, Währinger
Gürtel 18-20, A-1090 Vienna, Austria

Marie-Pierre Mayeur
Resident, Department of Surgery, Centre Alexis Vautrin, Avenue de Bourgogne, 54511
Vandoeuvre les Nancy, Cedex, France

Jose L. Monrós-Lliso   MD
Consultant, Department of Urology, Instituto Valenciano de Oncología, C/- Prof.
Beltran Baguena, 19, 46009 Valencia, Spain

Isabelle Pouchard
Resident, Centre Hospitalier Lyon-Sud, 69495 Pièrre-Benite, Cedex, France

Sidney B. Radomski   MD FRCS(C)
Assistant Professor, Department of Surgery, Division of Urology, University of Toronto,
The Toronto Hospital, Western Division, Toronto, Canada

Jose V. Ricós-Torrent   MD
Consultant, Department of Urology, Instituto Valenciano de Oncología, C/- Prof.
Beltran Baguena, 19, 46009 Valencia, Spain

Klaus Rüdiger   MD
Urologist, Schiffstrasse 9, 79098, Freiburg, Germany

Anne Schwander-Lesur   MD
Senior Consultant, Gynaecology Department, Centre Alexis Vautrin, Avenue de
Bourgogne, 54511 Vandoeuvre les Nancy, Cedex, France

Francesco P. Selvaggi   MD
Professor and Chairman of Urology, Chair of Urology 'R', University of Bari,
Policlinico PzaG. Cesare II, 70 124 Bari, Italy

Eduardo Solsona   MD

Head of Department, Department of Urology, Instituto Valenciano de Oncología, C/-Prof. Beltran Baguena, 19, 46009 Valencia, Spain

Horst Sommerkamp   MD

Professor and Chairman, Department of Urology, University Hospital, D-79106, Freiburg, Germany

Richard T. Turner-Warwick   CBE MD FRCP FRCS

Emeritus Surgeon, Institute of Urology, The Middlesex Hospital, Mortimer Street, London W1N 8AA, UK

Ulrich W. F. Wetterauer   MD

Associate Professor, Department of Urology, University Hospital, D-79106, Freiburg, Germany

Richard D. Williams   MD

Professor and Head, Department of Urology, The University of Iowa College of Medicine, Room 3251 RCP, 200 Hawkins Drive, Iowa City, IA, 52242-1089, USA

Preface

At the 22nd SIU Congress in Seville, the membership voted for a plenary session entitled 'Urological Complications of Pelvic Surgery and Radiotherapy' to be included in the programme to be held at the 23rd Congress in Sydney, Australia. This text is a collection of the Reporters' presentations, selected manuscripts requested from various presenters and invited manu-scripts to complete the subject matter. We have not really focused on the complications of radical prostatectomy and lymphadenectomy which were covered elsewhere at the Congress. These chapters are the work of experienced and knowledgeable urological surgeons and colleagues in radiation oncology. This text is intended to be a practically useful addition to the urologist's library.

The qualification and quantification of complications or side effects of all treatments, not just surgical, have become increasingly important. Surgeons have always attempted to describe outcome in terms of the desired results of treatment and have usually included the potential undesirable effects. The more recent focus on continued quality improvement and cost-effectiveness/benefit has sharpened the focus. Payors now want to known the ultimate cost of each treatment which naturally includes the cost to manage any potential side effect. Not only do we need better data on the true incidence of these side effects but we need to know how best to manage them in an effective way. The literature is replete with reports of short term follow-up but these are often from centres of excellence rather than based on a community experience. Tumour registries and other traditional data collection have not provided good information from broader population experience.

Centralization of data from inpatient care in some countries such as Canada and in many health maintenance organizations is providing a source for much higher quality information. Ironically, this is not being generated by the practitioners of medicine but rather the financial managers. In some jurisdictions, surgeons are being asked to provide total care of a presenting diagnosis including any complications that may arise for a pre-determined fee. This type of calculation is quite foreign to traditional medical practice and is a tremendous stimulant to accurate reporting including long term follow-up. Fortunately, surgeons perform many procedures that have a long history. In many ways they have an advantage over medical and radiation oncology colleagues. For example, it is relatively recently that we have recognized the increased incidence of secondary malignancies in some cancer survivors cured by chemotherapy.

Dr Dick Williams, who is the Rubin H. Flocks Chairman of the Department of Urology at the University of Iowa, has focused on the acute and longer term complications of pelvic surgery as they involve the bladder and prostate including fistula, pelvic abscess and continence and impotence. This overview includes an up-to-date list of references that will be very useful in pursuing more detail. In the work-day of the urological surgeon she/he is called upon to assist colleagues performing gynaecological and colorectal surgery when they encounter complications. Dr Williams describes the management of intra-operative injuries to the urinary tract as well as the range of possibilities when a fistula is recognized post-operatively. The traditional delay of 6–12 weeks or even longer to close a fistula is being modified and earlier surgery seems to be successful if inflammation has subsided. Certainly our patients appreciate an early closure. The percutaneous drainage of pelvic abscesses is now widely practised with a high rate of success. Not only has the incidence of abscess decreased but the morbidity rate has been dramatically reduced by this less invasive procedure. It can be accomplished quickly and with local anaesthetic in even a very ill patient. Urinary incontinence has many iatrogenic causes in addition to fistula, including neuropathy and pre-existent but undetected causes. Similarly, obstruction due to bladder neck contracture can occur. There is a useful discussion of lymphocoeles and impotence which is addressed in more detail by Dr Radomski and Dr Liquornik in Chapter 9. Dr Williams' contribution is a readable review of problems that we see regularly (fortunately with decreasing frequency) that we can refer to as needed.

Professor Francesco Selvaggi, Professor of Urology at the University of Bari, Italy and colleagues Dr Battaglia and Dr Cormio (from Helsinki University) have reviewed the ureteral complications of pelvic surgery and radiotherapy. This is an exhaustive and extensively referenced review with a careful compilation of their own experience including the important issue of prevention and diagnosis. The stratification of ureteral injuries by prognostic factors is useful. This systematizes the anecdotal experience that many of us have had. Thoughtful studies of ureteral stents are included as well as a discussion of techniques to improve results where there is inadequate ureteral length. These procedures have always fascinated surgeons but individuals rarely have a large experience to refine. We are indebted to Professor Selvaggi for this contribution, parts of which have been published in the peer reviewed literature and are referenced.

Professor Klaus Bandhauer from the Klinik für Urologie, Kantonsspital, St Gallen in Switzerland has reviewed the complications of ureteroscopy and current techniques of managing ureteral calculi, endo-urological management of UPJ obstruction, tumours and dilatation of the ureter. He goes on to a very clear discussion of the issues surrounding laparoscopic pelvic lymphadenectomy.

Dr Eduardo Solsona, Servicio de Urologia, Funçaçion Instituto Valenciano de Oncologia and colleagues have undertaken a truly monumental review of urological complications of pelvic radiotherapy. He clearly has a grasp of the subject and wide experience. The bibliography is particularly complete and useful.

Professor Nabil Bissada, Professor of Urology and the Chief of Urologic Oncology at the Medical University of South Carolina with colleague, Dr Johnson, has further elaborated on the management of fistulae following radiation which can cause very difficult problems. Fortunately, refinement of the dosimetry of radiotherapy has reduced this complication. Controversy remains regarding the potential for closure of these fistulae in heavily irradiated tissue. Many surgeons, myself included, are reluctant to attempt a primary closure even where healthy tissue can be interposed. Urinary diversion may be the preferred option. He recognizes the need for increased vascularity at the fistula site. The various flap techniques are clearly described and there is a good, up-to-date list of references.

Dr Oliver Hakenberg of the Division of Urology, University Hospital, Albert Ludwigs University of Freiburg, Germany, elaborates on the issues of urinary tract damage following radiotherapy for cervical carcinoma. In the short interval of two years, his unit saw 16 cases which are reviewed in the context of a thorough review of the literature that is very well referenced and should provide the most current publication on the subject.

Mr Chris Chapple of Central Sheffield University Hospital in the United Kingdom, and colleague Mr Richard Turner-Warwick, have carried this a step further with a discussion of the 'frozen pelvis'. Several cases are used to review the surgical principles and management of severe radiation injuries. These cases are rare but daunting and many of us should be reluctant to undertake this type of surgery, without prior training and experience. There is no question that these authors are master technicians working with a large population base that has concentrated this experience.

Dr Veronique Beckendorf of the Department of Radiotherapy at the Centre Alexis Vautrin in Nancy, France, has reported the results of a prospective study performed by the French radiation oncologists to assess sexual function and dysfunction after radiotherapy for carcinoma of the prostate. Many of the relevant issues including accurate measurement of pre-treatment function apply to the side effects of radiation therapy. Sexual dysfunction after the treatment of cervical carcinoma is not commonly appreciated by urologists and is discussed in some detail. This succinct review is also well referenced.

Dr Sidney Radomski and his colleague Dr Liquornik of the Division of Urology, University of Toronto, Canada have reviewed erectile function after pelvic surgery. While most patients undergoing surgery are in the older age group and are traditionally prepared to sacrifice sexual function, we have learned that it is actually a very important concern that is not always fully shared with the surgeon. Drs Radomski and Liquornik review the physiology of erection and detail the impact of the common surgical procedures in the pelvis and retroperitoneum. The management is detailed and thoroughly referenced. This chapter is a nice compliment to Dr Beckendorf's review of the effects of radiation therapy.

Finally, Professor Ulrich Maier and colleagues Dr Madersbacher and Professor Marberger of the Department of Urology at the University of Vienna, Austria have produced an interesting discussion of the urologic complications of renal transplantation. Urologists have varying degrees of involvement in renal transplantation. While historically initiating the procedure, transplantation departments and services have developed staffed by surgeons trained in transplantation. Regardless of the degree of involvement of the urologist at the time of transplantation the long term complications are usually managed by urologists with principles developed from non-transplantation surgery. This review of 21 patients from an experience of 1450 renal transplants is thorough. It addresses the most common and frequently difficult problems that we face. The very high success rate (90%) is a benchmark for the rest of us involved in this treatment.

I for one will value this book as a useful reference text in my library to reach for when I am thinking about the next patient that I am asked to see with a complication of pelvic radiation or surgery.

Michael A. S. Jewett

Urological complications of pelvic surgery

1

R. D. Williams

Introduction

Complications of pelvic surgery involving the lower urinary tract commonly emanate from surgery on the urinary tract itself; however, gynaecological surgery and colorectal surgery also account for a significant number of surgical problems. This chapter is limited to complications regarding the bladder, prostate, seminal vesicles and posterior urethra.

The complications relating to urological surgery can be divided into those occurring at the time of surgery, or immediately thereafter, and those delayed for several days. Acute complications include haemorrhage and urine leakage. Delayed complications include abscess formation; lymphocoeles, fistulae from the bladder or urethra to the vagina, rectum or skin; bladder neck contractures; incontinence; urethral stricture; and impotence. Complications arising from gynaecological surgery that occur acutely are primarily bladder lacerations, and those delayed include vesicovaginal and vesicourethral fistulae, and incontinence. Colorectical surgery can be complicated by vesical or prostatic laceration, resulting in vesicorectal or urethral–rectal fistulae. Incontinence, urinary retention and/or impotence may also occur in male patients following colorectal surgery.

Acute bladder complications

Laceration

In females this most common acute bladder injury occurs during abdominal hysterectomy. The bladder may be directly injured during dissection of the cervical cuff and proximal vagina, or it may be caught in a clamp placed across the proximal vagina at the resection of the distal cervix. Prevention, by careful dissection of the posterior bladder wall away from the anterior vaginal wall, is crucial. If a laceration is noted, an immediate two-layer closure using an absorbable suture is preferred. If serosal or peritoneal tissue is available, a third layer of closure may be useful. Catheter irrigation of the bladder to ensure a watertight closure and the use of intravenous indigo-carmine to eliminate a concomitant ureteral injury would be prudent. A urethral catheter should be left in place for 5–7 days. In a previously irradiated patient, an omental patch over the bladder closure should be considered. A suction drain overlying tissues near, but not at, the closure will be helpful for 2–3 days and can be removed when the drainage is minimal. If drainage persists, a drainage fluid creatinine concentration higher than that of the serum will prove the fluid to be urine. If the drainage fluid value is similar to that of serum, the fluid can be assumed to be peritoneal or lymphatic.

Bladder laceration also occurs in females during stress incontinence surgery or during vaginal hysterectomy.[1–3] The bladder is closed using the principles previously described. Vaginal closure requires more certainty of a watertight closure and separation of the vaginal and bladder closures, if possible, as no extravesical drain is left in place. It is important to make sure that the ureters are not involved. Recently, multiple urinary tract injuries have been described during laparoscopic hysterectomy.[4] Bladder laceration during colorectal surgery is approached in a similar manner for male or female patients.

Haemorrhage

Intravesical haemorrhage from an acute bladder laceration can be due to the presence of a larger laceration than initially recognized with an in-complete closure. Although this is unlikely, if it occurs transurethral fulguration may be the most prudent approach. Bladder irrigation with solutions such as alum, prostaglandins and formalin have been described but are not recommended in the acute situation; these methods are generally more suitable for haemorrhage associated with radiation cystitis or as a complication of systemic cyclophosphamide use.

Delayed bladder complications

Vesicovaginal fistula

In healthy women who have bladder injuries closed as previously described, subsequent complications are uncommon. In patients who are diabetic, or who have had previous pelvic irradiation or pelvic surgery, failure of the primary closure or development of a delayed fistula may occur.[5–7] An unnoticed bladder injury during hysterectomy, due to crush by a clamp or inclusion of the bladder by a vaginal suture, is most often the cause of a vesicovaginal fistula. In developing countries a more common cause is prolonged or difficult labour. In the United States today, vesicovaginal fistula is a less common problem, following less than 1% of hysterectomies.[6,8] Fistula formation occurs more commonly from an abdominal than a vaginal approach. The patient usually notes vaginal drainage 5 days to 2 weeks after surgery. Occasionally, prolonged urinary catheter drainage and/or fulguration of a small fistula will result in spontaneous closure, but, more commonly, definitive surgical closure will be necessary.[9–11] In patients with a radiation-induced fistula, hyperbaric oxygen as an adjunct to surgery to promote healing may prove beneficial.[12]

Surgical repair of a vesicovaginal fistula can be accomplished from a vaginal or abdominal approach. Timing is still controversial, although most surgeons who carry out this procedure frequently are now of the opinion that such fistulae should be repaired soon after they are discovered.[6] If infection is present in the adjacent tissues, a delay of several months may be appropriate.

The vaginal approach is preferred by many surgeons and can be done using many different methods, but all make use of similar principles of wide separation of vaginal and bladder mucosa with at least a two-layer closure of bladder and separate closure of the vagina. The vaginal closure can be done simply by using either a flap of vagina (Raz), or by transposition of one labial fat pad (Martius), the latter being particularly helpful in recurrent, difficult or tenuous repairs.[6,13,14] Large fistulae, or those with prior radiation, may require the use of myofascial or myocutaneous flaps from the perineum or thigh.[15,16] In general, the success rate with a vesicovaginal fistula repair in a previously non-irradiated or non-operated pelvis is over 90%. Closure of urethrovaginal fistulae is accomplished using the same principles.[17,18]

Patients with previous infection, pelvic radiation or multiple perineal procedures may benefit from an anterior abdominal approach.[12,19] The posterior bladder wall is separated from the vagina down to the fistula with, or without, a longitudinal bladder incision. A two-layer closure of the bladder and vagina is separated by an omental interposition. This approach has been found to be successful in up to 95% of patients. Alternatives for bladder closure include the use of a mucosa-free intestinal graft or peritoneal flap.[16,20] Recently, a laparoscopic approach to vesicovaginal fistula repair was described.[21] On the very rare occasions when multiple attempts at fistula closure have failed, urinary diversion may be necessary.[22]

Vesicouterine fistula

Vesicouterine fistulae are rare and most often caused by trauma, primarily during a caesarean section or prolonged childbirth.[11,23] Symptoms usually include cyclic haematuria or vaginal urinary incontinence. Diagnosis can be made by hysterography or cystography. The treatment can be hysterectomy and routine bladder closure in appropriate individuals. If the uterus is to be maintained, primary closure may require an abdominal approach, due to the high position of the cervix and the desirability of interposing omentum between the closures.

Enterovesical fistula

Enterovesical fistulae are most commonly secondary to inflammatory bowel disease or colorectal cancer. Iatrogenic surgical causes are often coincident in patients with bowel cancer treated with prior radiation or complicated by infection. The classic symptoms of suprapubic pain,

3

tenesmus and frequency with dysuria are common, as is pneumaturia, faecaluria and recurrent urinary tract infection. Diagnosis is made occasionally by examination of the urine after oral charcoal ingestion but more commonly by cystoscopy, where a herald patch is seen in 80% or more of cases.[24] A barium enema and/or a cystogram defines the fistula less commonly than expected, and computed tomography (CT) has now become the diagnostic modality of choice.[25,26] Ultrasonography and magnetic resonance imaging (MRI) have their proponents as well.[27] Although conservative treatment including bladder drainage, low-residue diet and/or intravenous hyperalimentation may allow spontaneous cure of some enterovesical fistulae, surgical repair is the general requirement.[28] Initial management of an acute iatrogenic enterovesical fistula may require temporary bowel diversion, i.e. ileostomy or colostomy, to allow inflammation to subside, followed by a definitive repair of the fistula and simultaneous reapproximation of the bowel.

The site of an iatrogenic enterovesical fistula is dependent on the pelvic surgery performed. After direct bladder surgery it would be unusual for the rectum to be injured; however, transvesical surgery on the seminal vesicles could result in rectal injury. The sigmoid could be injured or its blood supply compromised during pelvic surgery; however, this would be unlikely to produce a bladder fistula. A small bowel fistula following augmentation cystoplasty is possible but uncommon. Recent reports of a colovesical fistula after laparoscopic hernia repair raises concern that this new form of surgery may provide new statistics on surgical pelvic injury.[29]

Vesicocutaneous fistula

Vesicocutaneous leaks after bladder surgery are uncommon but can provide a substantial challenge for treatment. In general, if adequate bladder drainage from a urethral and/or a suprapubic catheter is present as well as a percutaneous drain (Penrose or suction drain), most leaks will spontaneously heal with time. If a drain is not previously placed, an ultrasound-guided perivesical drain may suffice. If persistent drainage and a true fistula develop, surgical correction may be required. Excision of the tract with debridement and closure of well-vascularized bladder edges is necessary. Usually these are anterior or lateral wall problems; however, the fistula may involve a ureter and thus the appropriate diagnostic steps should be taken before the repair. In patients with previous pelvic radiation therapy or pelvic infection, a vascularized flap of rectus muscle, demucosalized small intestine or omentum may be required to provide adequate healing.

Pelvic abscess

Abscess formation complicating pelvic surgery is less common today. Prophylactic antibiotics given perioperatively in patients with sterile urine, as well as preoperative bowel preparation, account for the low frequency. The most common procedures resulting in pelvic abscess involve concomitant bowel surgery such as augmentation cystoplasty or radical cystectomy with urinary diversion. Although most abscesses are first evident around postoperative day 5, many may be delayed for several weeks. Initially, the abscess may be difficult to diagnose, in that symptoms may be non-specific, such as malaise, low-grade fever, diarrhoea or ileus. The diagnosis is occasionally made when the abscess drains spontaneously through the vagina or male urethra. Preferably the diagnosis can be made by either pelvic ultrasonography showing a mass of variable echogenicity displacing bowel and/or bladder, or pelvic CT showing a medium-attenuation mass without contrast enhancement. The most common organisms are bowel flora, although in debilitated patients or those with compromised immunity fungal infections are not unusual.

Treatment in the past was by open incision and drainage—a procedure that still has great merit. Alternatively, and preferably now, percutaneous drainage can be done by the use of ultrasound- or CT-guided tube placement. This approach is highly effective (80%) in non-loculated abscesses. The percutaneous approach can be anteriorly, through the abdomen, or from the perineum or adjacent to the sacrum. In general, irrigation, with or without antibiotics, is unnecessary. If percutaneous drainage is unsuccessful, open drainage will be required.

Vesical dysfunction

Incontinence is rarely a complication of bladder surgery unless the rhabdosphincter is damaged. This may occur in male patients undergoing an abdominal–perineal colon resection and rarely following an anterior resection, or proctocolectomy, or in females after an abdominal hysterectomy. Because the majority of these patients do not have preoperative bladder function studies, it is not known whether the condition was present before surgery. The types of injuries encountered can vary, such as somatic (temporary), parasympathetic or sympathetic lesion.[30] The abdominal–perineal resection group tend to have a temporary condition. Long term, those patients with a substantial lesion exhibit stable dysfunction consisting of a large bladder capacity and detrusor hypoactivity suggestive of persistent parasympathetic denervation. A flaccid bladder neck will occur in many of these patients, suggesting sympathetic denervation as well. Treatment consists primarily of intermittent catheterization. A prosthetic artificial sphincter may be required if incontinence persists.

Acute prostatic complications

Laceration
The prostate can be damaged during pelvic surgery, albeit rarely. The

most frequent procedure accounting for prostate laceration is an abdominal–perineal resection. In general, a prostatic laceration is an inconsequential event unless the prostatic urethra is entered. If this is recognized, the urethra can be closed with absorbable sutures and a catheter left indwelling for 7–10 days; if it is unrecognized, a prostatorectal or prostatoperineal fistula may develop and can prove quite difficult to repair. Initially, if the fistula is small, transurethral fulguration and long-term catheter drainage may allow healing; if it is not small, transperineal closure may be required, with consideration of implementing a vascularized perineal muscle flap.

Haemorrhage

The rich arterial blood supply of the prostate is infrequently damaged during pelvic surgery. The arteries are branches of the inferior vesical and enter the prostate laterally just distal to the bladder neck. The venous drainage of the prostate and urethra is highly variable, with numerous collaterals and often very large vessels that are unforgiving to the novice pelvic surgeon. The dorsal vein of the penis drains toward the apex of the prostate where it joins Santorini's plexus, which fans out over the prostate. Injury to these vessels occurs during radical cystectomy, radical prostatectomy or simple open prostatectomy. The bleeding can be significant and rapid. The primary tools necessary to deal with prostatic venous bleeding are exposure and anatomical knowledge. In most instances the dorsal vein can be encircled directly anterior to the urethra by a free tie placed by a right-angle clamp above the urethra or a stick tie using a 5/8 curved needle directly under the pubis and above the urethra. If this is unsuccessful, better exposure can be obtained by incising the rectus muscle attachments to the pubis and flexing the operating table to expose the pelvis. If necessary, part or all of the pubic symphysis can be resected to expose the entire vein.

When removing the prostate, with or without bladder resection, if dorsal vein bleeding is hard to control, the urethra should be transected carefully and quickly, a Foley catheter placed in the urethra and the balloon inflated to 10 ml. Gentle traction is then placed on the catheter while the prostate/bladder is removed. The dorsal vein can then be oversewn subsequently, with better vision in a relatively empty pelvis. Usually, with the prostate removed, the bleeding decreases and, if the bladder neck is to be anastomosed to the urethra, securing the vesicourethral anastomotic sutures, with or without perineal approximation sutures (Vest), compresses the offending veins. If the bleeding is only venous and the anastomosis is well approximated, abdominal pressure from the awake patient with some postoperative pain will further compress the veins and any remaining minor bleeding will cease. A suction drain in the pelvis (not directly against the anastomosis) will adequately drain blood and urine and, usually, adequately warn of persistent haemorrhage. In very rare and severe instances, vaginal gauze packing in the pelvis can be used to compress tightly the venous bleeding. The patient's wound is closed with the packing exiting from the lower portion of the incision. The packing is removed 2–3 days later over 24–48 h. This approach can be life saving in extreme circumstances.

Urine leak

Immediately postoperatively from a radical prostatectomy or open prostatectomy there may be a substantial urine leak through the suprapubic or perineal drain. Although it is imperative that the leakage stops, it is not an emergency situation unless no urine drainage is evident from the urethral catheter or there is the possibility of a ureteral injury. Initially, it is important to determine that the catheter is in the bladder and draining appropriately, as, on occasion, the catheter will be displaced outside the urinary tract. If urine is draining from the catheter and it irrigates, it is unlikely to be misplaced; however, a cystogram can readily identify its position. Obviously, if it is not in the bladder it must be replaced. In this situation, occasionally, simple removal of the catheter and replacement is successful; thus, one cautious attempt at catheterization is reasonable. Flexible cystoscopy with passage of a guidewire and catheter over the wire is a second possibility. It may be safest to reoperate immediately, to replace the catheter under direct vision and to repair the anastomosis if necessary.

If the catheter is confirmed to be in place, an initial few hours of urine leakage from the drain is not bothersome and often will recede as the patient has better pain control and is treated for bladder spasms. If a suction drain has been used, persistent drainage is treated by discontinuing suction and placing the tubing on gravity drainage (not clamped) into a closed bag. Suction should be re-established for a few minutes every few hours. Slight advancement of the suction drain or Penrose drain (away from the anastomosis) may be required if the drainage does not cease. Usually, within a few hours to a few days, the drainage ceases. It would be prudent to monitor the creatinine level in the drainage fluid if it persists for an extended period, to determine whether the drainage continues to contain urine. The drain is removed when the collection is less than 30–40 ml every 8 h. Persistent urinary leakage, particularly if the volume is one-half or more of the urinary output, could signify other major problems, such as vesicourethral anastomotic disruption or ureteral injury; appropriate radiographic studies, such as a cystogram, an intravenous urogram or pelvic CT with contrast, should be obtained in these circumstances.

Delayed prostatic complications

Pelvic lymphocoele

Pelvic lymphocoeles do not commonly present symptomatically after pelvic surgery, yet they occur much more often than they are detected. Most lymphocoeles will be small and self-contained, and cause no symptoms. Most commonly, lymphocoeles occur after renal transplantation or the pelvic lymph node dissection accompanying radical prostatectomy, radical cystoprostatectomy, ovarian tumour resection or abdominal hysterectomy. The mere presence of a lymphocoele does not require treatment. They are usually asymptomatic, but in large lymph collections can cause pelvic pain, abdominal distension, urinary frequency, ureteral obstruction, iliac vein compression, and/or lower-extremity oedema. The diagnosis is made from a pelvic ultrasound or CT. A postoperative imaging study on an asymptomatic patient may show a lymphocoele but, if no sequelae are noted, it should remain undisturbed. There is evidence that lymphocoeles are more common in patients on subcutaneous heparin for deep vein thrombosis prophylaxis but occur infrequently when meticulous occlusion of lymphatic channels by suture or clip ligation is accomplished.

Symptomatic lymphocoeles can be drained percutaneously by ultrasound or CT guidance with a tube left in place for 24–48 h and then removed. Care must be taken not to infect the lymphocoele. If the collection continues to be symptomatic a second attempt at percutaneous drainage may be helpful but, if a symptomatic lymphocoele persists, marsupialization of the lymphocoele into the peritoneal cavity by an open or laparoscopic technique will be necessary. During these operations care must be taken not to injure neighbouring organs, such as ureters, colon or bladder, that may be immediately adjacent to the lymphocoele capsule. The most significant problem occurs when a lymphocoele becomes secondarily infected. Systemic antibiotics may be successful for treatment, but percutaneous or open drainage with antibiotic irrigation may be required to treat the condition effectively, particularly those occurring after renal transplantation.

Bladder neck contracture

The incidence of bladder neck contracture after radical prostatectomy is approximately 10%.[31] In most instances the patient complains of a slow stream that can be documented by uroflow studies. The diagnosis can be made by a retrograde urethrogram or, preferably, by flexible cystoscopy. Very short (< 0.5 cm) strictures can be dilated by catheter dilators or Amplatz dilators; the long-term success is more than 90%. For persistent and/or longer strictures single dilation will not usually suffice. Once dilation has been achieved, intermittent catheterization over a 6–12 week period may prove to be curative; more often, a transurethral incision using a cold or hot knife or laser will be required to restore normal voiding. There is a danger that incontinence will result; however, judicious cuts proximal to the external sphincter are relatively safe. The patient may have incontinence briefly but regain continence shortly thereafter. There is also a danger of a rectal laceration that can be obviated by incisions at three and nine o'clock, avoiding the six o'clock position. Intermittent catheterization for a few weeks after a transurethral incision will allow the bladder neck to heal satisfactorily without restricture.

Incontinence

The incontinence rate after radical prostate surgery ranges from 19 to 40% in the literature.[32–34] The definition of incontinence in these reports varies widely and thus the true incidence is difficult to state definitively. Using the definition that total incontinence means 'wet all the time— never dry', only 1–2% of men after a radical perineal or retropubic prostatectomy are totally incontinent. Stress incontinence, meaning 'urine leakage on abdominal straining, lifting, participating in sports, etc., requiring pads (more than a few drops)' occurs in 20–50% of patients. More than one-half of the patients will have a few drops of leakage on straining, particularly in the late afternoon, but not requiring pads. In general, work-up of the stress-incontinent patients will show an intrinsic bladder (or, more commonly, urethral sphincter) abnormality that may have predated prostate surgery. The totally incontinent patients will show a very short membranous urethra and an intrinsic external sphincter insufficiency that is probably iatrogenic.

Treatment of the totally incontinent patient with pharmacotherapy such as anticholinergic drugs will be unsuccessful. An artificial sphincter is the only successful method, short of bladder neck reconstruction or urinary diversion, to provide continence.[35] For stress incontinence, Teflon (or, more recently, collagen) submucosal transurethral injections have become useful. In selected patients without substantial bladder neck scar tissue these injections are 60–80% successful at reducing or eliminating stress incontinence in short-term studies.

Impotence

Discovery of the anatomy of the nerves responsible for erection is one of the more important findings in recent urological history. The surgical procedure for sparing these nerves during radical prostatectomy with or without cystectomy is a urological milestone, particularly for younger men. In properly selected patients without the likelihood of tumour extension beyond the prostate capsule, a potency-sparing procedure is appropriate. The success depends on the surgeon's experience. Walsh describes more than 80% efficacy in his highly selected series of younger men. There is sparse documentation other than anecdotal evidence of potency in any reported series. Recent patient surveys (patient questionnaires) report a much lower potency rate, averaging 5–20% full erection.[33,36,37] No adequate prospective study of patients' potency before and after surgery has been reported.

Injury to the nerves responsible for erection can occur during rectal surgery, prostatic or seminal vesicle surgery and cystoprostatectomy. The principles of nerve-sparing surgery are the same in all these procedures. The potency following rectal surgery is reported to be more than 80%;[38] that after nerve-sparing radical cystectomy without urethrectomy is approximately 50%, and with urethrectomy it is 20–30%.

Management of impotence after radical pelvic surgery depends on many variables.[34,37,39,40] Many patients may be uninterested and thus should have information only offered. Yohimbine is not useful. Vacuum erection devices seem unaesthetic but are often preferred by patients, given all the choices. Over 60% of patients who initiate the use of a vacuum device continue to use it successfully. Penile injections of vasoactive agents are quite successful but patients are put off by the idea of injections and the drop-out rate after initial enthusiasm is high. The use of penile prostheses has declined substantially in the United States. Currently, the patients who are younger than 60 and quite motivated seem to prefer inflatable prostheses but, overall, the number of post-radical prostatectomy patients requesting prostheses is relatively few.

Urethrorectal fistula

This is one of the most feared complications of radical prostatectomy or orthotopic continent diversion after a radical cystectomy. Fortunately, the incidence is less than 1%. Previous radiation therapy; intraoperative rectal laceration; and previous rectal, vesical or prostatic surgery, all predispose to this complication. Treatment of a postoperative urethral vesical anastomotic stricture can also lead to a urethrorectal fistula.

Diagnosis is usually not difficult as the patient complains of a decrease in urine output through the penis and a simultaneous increase in fluid per rectum. The fistula is usually evident several days to weeks after surgery. A cystogram, CT with contrast or cystoscopy are all effective methods of documenting the presence of a fistula.

Treatment by fulguration of a small fistula may be successful. Diversion of the urine by a suprapubic cystostomy may also be helpful. Persistent fistulae will require definitive surgical repair. A temporary diverting colostomy may be, but is not always, necessary. Faecaluria with urinary infection would indicate the need for colostomy. Methods for surgical repair include retropubic with an omental interposition, perineal with the possible interposition of a gracilis or other muscle flap, transcoccygeal (Kraske) with a possible gluteal flap, or a transrectal sphincter procedure. Of these, the former is the least and the latter the most desirable procedure. In non-irradiated tissue the success rate of these procedures is more than 90%.

The major principles in managing urological complications of pelvic surgery are primarily as follows: prevention; early recognition; extensive diagnostic evaluation of all possible accompanying injuries; and choosing the most definitive treatment option first, without compromise.

References

1. Elkins T. Surgery for the obstetric vesicovaginal fistula: a review of 100 operations in 82 patients. Am J Obstet Gynecol 1994; 170: 1108–1120
2. Goodwin W, Scardino P T. Vesicovaginal and ureterovaginal fistulas: a summary of 25 years of experience. J Urol 1980; 123: 370–374
3. Hedlund H, Lindstedt E. Urovaginal fistulas: 20 years of experience with 45 cases. J Urol 1987; 137: 926–928
4. Kadar N, Lemerling C. Urinary tract injuries during laparoscopically assisted hysterectomy: causes and prevention. Am J Obstet Gynecol 1994; 170: 47–48
5. Arrowsmith S D. Genitourinary reconstruction in obstetric fistulas. J Urol 1994; 152: 403–406
6. Little N A, Juma S, Raz S. Vesicovaginal fistulas. Semin Urol 1989; 7: 78–85
7. Marshall V F. Vesicovaginal fistulas on one urological service. J Urol 1979; 121: 25–29
8. Tancer M L. The post-total hysterectomy (vault) vesicovaginal fistula. J Urol 1980; 123: 839–840
9. Molina L R, Lynne C M, Politano VA. Treatment of vesicouterine fistula by fulguration. J Urol 1989; 141: 1422–1423
10. Stovsky M D, Ignatoff J M, Blum M D et al. Use of electrocoagulation in the treatment of vesicovaginal fistulas. J Urol 1994; 152: 1443–1444
11. Thanos A, Pavlakis A J, Poulias I et al. Vesicouterine fistuli. Urology 1986; 28: 426–428
12. Velagapudi S R C, Pollack H W, Weiss J P. Acquired fistulas of the urinary tract. AUA Update Ser 1993; 12: 138–143
13. Margolis T, Elkins T E, Seffah J et al. Full-thickness martius grafts to preserve vaginal depth as an adjunct in the repair of large obstetric fistulas. Obstet Gynecol 1994; 84: 148–152
14. Raz S, Bregg K J, Nitti V W, Sussman E. Transvaginal repair of vesicovaginal fistula using a peritoneal flap. J Urol 1993; 150: 56–59
15. Palmer J A, Vernon C P, Cummings B J, Moffot F L. Gracilis myocutaneous flap for reconstructing perineal defects resulting from radiation and radical surgery. Can J Surg 1983; 26: 510–512
16. Salup R R, Julian T B, Liang M D et al. Closure of large post radiation vesicovaginal fistula with rectus abdominis myofascial flap. Urology 1994; 44: 130–131
17. Webster G E, Sihelnik S A, Stone A R. Urethrovaginal fistula: a review of the surgical management. J Urol 1984; 132: 460–462
18. Zimmern P, Schmidbauer C P, Leach G E, et al. Vesicovaginal and urethrovaginal fistulae. Semin Urol 1986; 4: 24–29
19. Kristensen J K, Lose G. Vesicovaginal fistulas: the transperitoneal repair revisited. Scand J Urol Nephrol 1994; 157: 101–105
20. Mráz J P, Sutorý M. An alternative in surgical treatment of post-irradiation vesicovaginal and rectovaginal fistulas: the seromuscular intestinal graft (patch). J Urol 1994; 151: 357–359
21. Nezhat C H, Nezhat F, Nezhat C, Rottenberg H. Laparoscopic repair of a vesicovaginal fistula. Obstet Gynecol 1994; 83: 899–901
22. Wan J, McGuire E J. Augmentation cystoplasty and closure of the urethra for the destroyed lower urinary tract. J Am Paraplegia Soc 1990; 13: 40–45
23. Virtanen H S, Mäkinen J I. Vesicocervical fistula—a rare cause of urinary incontinence. Eur J Obstet Gynecol Reprod Biol 1994; 57: 54–55
24. Lippert MC, Teates C D, Howards S S. Detection of enteric-urinary fistulas with a non-invasive quantitative method. J Urol 1984; 132: 1134–1136
25. Jarrett T W, Vaughn E D Jr. Accuracy of computerized tomography in the diagnosis of colovesical fistula secondary to diverticular disease. J Urol 1995; 153: 44–46

26. Narumi Y, Sato T, Kuriyama K et al. Computed tomographic diagnosis of enterovesical fistulae: barium evacuation method. Gastrointest Radiol 1988; 155: 331–335

27. Chen S S, Chou Y H, Tiu C M et al. Sonographic features of colovesical fistula. J Clin Ultrasound 1990; 18: 589–591

28. Moss R L, Ryan J A Jr. Management of enterovesical fistulas. Am J Surg 1990; 159: 514–517

29. Gray M R, Curtis J M, Elkington J S. Colovesical fistula after laparoscopic inguinal hernia repair. Br J Surg 1994; 81: 1213–1214

30. Yalla S V, Andriole G L. Vesicourethral dysfunction following pelvic visceral ablative surgery. J Urol 1984; 132: 503–509

31. Jønler M, Messing E M, Rhodes P R, Bruskewitz R C. Sequelae of radical prostatectomy. Br J Urol 1994; 74: 352–358

32. Braslis K G, Santa-Cruz C, Brickman A L, Soloway M S. Quality of life 12 months after radical prostatectomy. Br J Urol 1995; 75: 48–53

33. Chodak G W, Skinner M, Rukstalis D B et al. Patient-reported outcomes following radical prostatectomy performed at eight academic institutions. J Urol 1995; 153: 390A

34. Schover L R. Sexual rehabilitation after treatment for prostate cancer. Cancer 1993; 71: 1024–1030

35. Sullivan M P, Hutcheson J, Yalla S V. Management of incontinence following radical prostatectomy. Infect Urol 1995; 8: 46–56

36. Murphy G P, Mettlin C, Menck H et al. National patterns of prostate cancer treatment by radical prostatectomy: results of a survey by the American College of Surgeons Commission on Cancer. J Urol 1994; 152: 1817–1819

37. Pavone-Macaluso M. Are organ preservation and maintenance of sexual function compatible with optimal management of prostate cancer? (Editorial) Prog Clin Biol Res 1991; 370: 203–205

38. Enker W E. Potency, cure, and local control in the operative treatment of rectal cancer. Arch Surg 1992; 127: 1396–1402

39. Koraitim M, Khalil R. Preservation of urosexual functions after radical cystectomy. Urology 1992; 39: 117–121

40. Tomic R, Sjödin J G. Sexual function in men after radical cystectomy with or without urethrectomy. Scand J Urol Nephrol 1992; 26: 127–129

Ureteral complications of pelvic surgery

2

F. P. Selvaggi   M. Battaglia   L. Cormio

Introduction

Although the ureter is protected from injury by external agents by virtue of its elasticity and sheltered position, it is highly vulnerable during surgical procedures or radiotherapy performed in the pelvic area, owing to its close attachment to the peritoneum and proximity to major pelvic organs. Hence, the repair of iatrogenic injuries has assumed considerable importance in the 20th century with the development of advanced pelvic surgery and radiotherapy. In 1900, Wertheim[1] reported a 10% incidence of ureteral injuries following radical hysterectomy and, in 1920, Schmitz[2] reported the first case of ureteral stricture attributable to radiotherapy.

Interest in the ureteral complications of pelvic surgery and radiotherapy has recently revived, not because these have in fact changed but because new technology and materials are now available, while experience has allowed better insight on which to base the choice of treatment.

Definition, epidemiology and aetiology

By 'true complications' of pelvic surgery or radiotherapy is meant those whereby previously healthy ureters are damaged accidentally. The involuntary nature of the involvement provides the differential aetio-pathogenic basis compared, for example, with a ureteral perforation occurring during ureteral lithotripsy or fulguration of a papillary carcinoma, procedures that are performed on an already compromised organ.

In the authors' experience (Table 2.1) all kinds of pelvic surgery, with or without radiotherapy, can be at the origin of the former kind of ureteral injury.

The overall incidence of ureteral injuries following pelvic surgery and/or radiotherapy appears to be the same as when reported by Dowling and co-workers[3] at 0.5–1%. This is due to the fact that, although the incidence of ureteral injuries during major pelvic surgery has tended to decrease, owing to improved expertise, there is, on the other hand, an increased incidence of lesions during routine procedures, while new aetiological factors have arisen that also affect this figure.

Classic aetiological factors

Gynaecological and obstetric procedures

These probably remain the most frequent cause of ureteral injuries.

Aetiology*	No. of patients	Bilateral injury	No. of ureters	Site			Length			Type of injury				
				Upper	Middle	Lower	<2 cm	2–5 cm	>5 cm	Stricture	Avulsion	Reflux	Fistula	Radiotherapy
O/G	83	24	107	—	5	102	58	40	9	72	—	—	35	38
U	39	6	45	11	13	21	29	12	4	33	—	2	10	2
GS	15	—	15	—	7	8	11	3	1	5	—	—	10	—
O	1	—	1	—	—	1	—	—	1	—	1	—	—	—
ET	4	—	4	1	2	1	1	2	1	2	—	—	2	—
Total	142	30	172	12	27	133	99	57	16	112	1	2	57	40

Table 2.1. Ureteral injuries observed from June 1972 to August 1994
*O/G, obstetric/gynaecological; U, urological; GS, general surgical; O, orthopaedic surgical; ET, external trauma.

Solomons and co-workers[4] analysed 33 086 surgical procedures for benign and malignant lesions; ureteral injuries occurred in 0.8% of cases. In two recent retrospective series of 3185 and 1093 patients who had undergone obstetric or gynaecological procedures, the incidence of ureteral injury was 0.5 and 1.5%, respectively.[5,6]

Nearly two-thirds of these injuries occur during abdominal procedures, such as abdominal hysterectomy, abdominal oophorectomy, caesarean section and caesarean hysterectomy, while one-third occur during vaginal procedures, such as vaginal hysterectomy, vaginal oophorectomy, forceps delivery, and even abortion.[7] The reported incidence of ureteral injury due to caesarean section is 0.1%.[8] In two prospective studies the incidence of ureteral injury after hysterectomy for benign disease was 2.4 and 2.5%, respectively.[4,9] The incidence of ureteral injury after radical hysterectomy has remained constant at about 10% since Wertheim's time,[1] although variations from 5 to 30% have been reported in different series.[10,11]

The most common sites of injury to the ureter are at the level of the pelvic brim (where the ureter lies in close proximity to the ovarian vessels), at the level of the infundibulopelvic ligament (where it runs under the uterine artery) and at the level of the ureterovesical junction.[12] Risk factors include previous radiotherapy, previous operations in the pelvis, endometriosis, previous inflammatory pelvic disease, distorted anatomy of the region, and removal of the adnexa after previous hysterectomy.[13] Nevertheless, 75% of the ureteral injuries due to obstetric or gynaecological surgery occur during procedures described by the surgeon as 'uncomplicated'.[14]

General surgical procedures

Abdominal perineal resection is the general surgical procedure most frequently associated with ureteral injury, the incidence of such complications varying from 0.3 to 5.7% in different series.[15,16] The ureter may be injured during division of the mesosigmoid, of the lateral ligaments of the rectum, of the inferior mesenteric artery, or during retroperitonealization.[17,18] In the latter case, the ureteral injury may be the result of a certain loss of concentration on the part of the surgeon after the most difficult part of the procedure has been completed.

The left ureter is more likely to be injured due to its close proximity to the mesosigmoid;[16] to avoid this complication, more extensive isolation of the ureter has been suggested.

Inguinal herniorrhaphy[19] or removal of a retrocaecal appendix may rarely be responsible for ureteral injury.[20]

Vascular surgical procedures

Procedures such as sympathectomy and aorto-iliac or aortofemoral bypass surgery can also cause ureteral injuries. In a prospective study on 20 patients in whom intravenous urography (IVU) was performed 2 weeks and 12 months after aorto-iliac or aortofemoral surgery, the incidence of hydronephrosis was 20% at 2 weeks and 10% at 1-year follow-up.[21] In another prospective study, 181 kidneys in 93 patients who had undergone aortofemoral bypass surgery were examined by ultrasound at 1 week, 3 months and 1 year postoperatively. Mild to moderate hydronephrosis was found in 15 kidneys at 1-week follow-up and in only one kidney at 1-year follow-up.[22] Thus, it would seem that hydronephrosis occurring after aortofemoral bypass surgery is not uncommon but is rarely of clinical significance in the asymptomatic patient. In most cases it is due to extensive fibrotic reaction around the vascular graft.

Ureteral fistula after aortofemoral bypass surgery, conversely, is quite rare but always clinically significant. Reviewing 154 cases of ureteral obstruction after aortofemoral surgery, Blasco and Saladie[23] found that ureteral fistula had developed in 19 cases (12%) and that radiological signs of ureteral obstruction always preceded fistula formation.

Urological procedures

It is difficult to assess the true incidence of ureteral injuries attributable to urological procedures as, in most cases, the lesion is diagnosed intraoperatively and repaired immediately, without being recorded. This is particularly true of lesions that are caused by ureteroscopic procedures, which are discussed in a subsequent section.

The ureter may be injured in the course of excision of vesical diverticula, as well as during simple or radical prostatectomy.[24]

Radiotherapy

To date, ureteral injuries that are due to radiotherapy are infrequent. The reported incidence of ureteral strictures in patients treated with radiotherapy for carcinoma of the cervix is 1%.[25] However, this incidence rises to 5.3% in patients also subjected to open surgery[26] or prophylactic catheterization of the ureters.[27] Contrary to these clinical data, which suggest that the ureter is radioresistant, experimental studies have shown it to be the most radiosensitive abdominal organ as it tolerates only 20–25 Gy, much less than the dose usually administered.[28,29]

Ureteral obstruction following irradiation and surgery begins within 3–4 months, while ureteral obstruction following irradiation alone may occur within a period ranging from 6 months to 10 years.[30] Radiation injuries seem to occur 4–6 cm from the ureteral orifice at a point where the ureter crosses the broad ligament that corresponds to the point of highest radiation dosage. The histological changes seen in radiated ureters have been divided into three stages.[31] In the acute stage, seen immediately after irradiation, there is hyperaemia, oedema, and degeneration of the uroepithelium and endothelium. In the subacute stage there is progression of the epithelial and endothelial changes and the presence of an inflammatory infiltrate. Finally, in the chronic stage, endoarteritis obliterans develops, leading to decreased blood supply and consequent tissue atrophy.

In clinical practice, however, only a few patients treated with radiotherapy will develop a clinically significant complication, usually stricture. This would suggest that the effects of radiotherapy depend on the condition of the organ rather than on the radiotherapy itself, probably because a healthy ureter is able to repair mild damage.

New aetiological factors

The introduction of new techniques has led to the creation of new aetiological factors for ureteral injuries.

Ureteroscopy

Owing to its increasing use, ureteroscopy has become one of the leading causes of ureteral injuries. In 15 series totalling 1696 ureteroscopic procedures, injuries occurred in 9% (range 0–28%) of all procedures, and consisted of perforation of the ureter in 7% of cases, avulsion in 0.4% and postoperative stricture formation in 1.4%.[32] Although the proximal third of the ureter is more prone to injury because it has less muscle support and a thinner lining of mucosal cells than the distal ureter,[30] most injuries occur in the distal third of the ureter, where more procedures are performed.[33] Perforation may occur when forcing a passage, especially when negotiating kinks or strictures. Stricture may also result from a direct mucosal injury by the instrument. These injuries are discussed in chapter 3.

Orthopaedic surgery

Procedures such as arthrodesis of the hip joint and total hip replacement[34,35] have occasionally been reported to cause ureteral lesions.

Other procedures

Laparoscopic procedures such as laparoscopic sterilization,[36] laparoscopic fulguration of pelvic endometriosis[37] and laparoscopically assisted vaginal hysterectomy[38] may exceptionally cause ureteral injuries. Recently, even extracorporeal shock-wave lithotripsy,[39] oocyte recovery for in vitro fertilization[40] and CT-guided chemical sympathectomy[41] have been reported to cause ureteral injuries.

Prevention

Preoperative catheterization of the ureter was recommended in the past to prevent ureteral injuries due to gynaecological procedures,[42] as well as those due to general surgical procedures.[43] The experience gained over the years has shown that preoperative catheterization is not effective in preventing the trauma[44] and could even provoke it.[45,46]

The use of transilluminating ureteral stents has recently been advocated for preventing ureteral injuries during gynaecological procedures,[47] but does not seem to be effective. Conversely, careful identification of the ureter in the retroperitoneal area and, when necessary, judicious mobilization of the portion at risk before performing major gynaecological surgical procedures have proved to be effective in preventing ureteral injuries.[5,6,13]

Diagnosis

The experience gained over the last 20 years confirms the importance of the time of diagnosis. Unfortunately, the incidence of injuries diagnosed intraoperatively has not changed, although intraoperative identification offers the best results and allows immediate repair of the lesion, thus avoiding further procedures.[7,48]

Injuries due to ligation, devascularization or fulguration of the ureter are unlikely to be recognized intraoperatively. Even small ureteral sections often pass unrecognized at surgery as a small urine leak may easily resemble the normal tissue fluid. In unclear cases, intravenous administration of dyes such as methylene blue or indigo carmine represents a simple and effective method for verifying the presence of a small ureteral section. Similarly, intra-operative intravenous pyelography (IVP) may help to visualize ureteral ligation. When in doubt, even insertion of a ureteral catheter may be preferable to repairing an injury later.

More than 80% of ureteral injuries still present postoperatively.[49] Total ureteral obstruction due to ligation presents with severe flank pain, often associated with fever, nausea and vomiting. Postoperative anuria may be present in the case of bilateral ureteral injury. Partial ureteral obstruction due to devascularization or fulguration may or may not present with flank pain. In the latter case, functional exclusion of the kidney may occur in the absence of any symptom. Ureteral section or crushing results in urinary extravasation which leads within the first 10 postoperative days either to urinoma formation, if the urine remains confined in the retroperitoneum, or to the development of ureterocutaneous or ureterovaginal fistulae, if the urine finds a way out. Malaise, fever and vague gastrointestinal symptoms are often found in the case of urinoma; watery discharges from the wound or the vagina, conversely, occur in the case of fistulae. The watery discharge from the wound or the vagina can easily be identified as urine by determining the creatinine concentration of a small sample (urine has many times the creatinine concentration found in serum), or by intravenous injection of methylene blue or indigo carmine, which will appear in the urine as dark blue.[50]

Ultrasonography

Apart from the clinical signs, ultrasonography has become a fundamental tool in the diagnosis of ureteral injuries. Although not highly specific, it is the simplest and least invasive method for investigating a suspected ureteral injury, displaying, at the patient's bedside, the presence of hydronephrosis or of retroperitoneal fluid collection (urinoma) attributable to urinary extravasation.

Intravenous urography

IVU is essential to determine the site, kind and length of the ureteral injury. It also offers valuable information on kidney function, as well as on possible coexisting or pre-existing pathologies of the homolateral or contralateral kidney. Cystograms and voiding cystourethrograms at the end of IVU may be useful to rule out vesicovaginal fistulae and to evaluate the status of the bladder before a bladder elongation technique is considered.

Retrograde pyelography

This remains the best tool for investigating the ureteral tract distal to the lesion. Although this information may be of little importance in open surgical repair, it becomes of major importance when planning endo-urological treatment, as it completes the work-up and may constitute the first step of such treatment.

Computed tomography (CT scan) and magnetic resonance imaging (MRI)

These can be used to search for urinoma or abscesses,[51] but their main role is in ruling out possible recurrence of tumour.

Renal radionuclide scanning

This may be necessary in the case of strictures diagnosed several months after the aetiological trauma, to determine whether the renal function is worthy of salvage and to monitor it after surgical correction.

Urodynamic investigations

These have recently gained further importance as a means of differentiating between hydronephrosis due to ureteral obstruction and hydronephrosis due to bladder denervation after major pelvic surgery, and of evaluating detrusor and sphincter function before any surgical reconstructive procedure is chosen.

Current management

The management of ureteral injuries presents a challenge, owing to the rarity of the condition, the number of therapeutic options available and, in particular, the lack of prognostic factors directing the therapeutic choice.

It is common opinion[7] that ureteral injuries recognized during surgery should be repaired immediately. Short injuries of the middle third of the ureter can be managed with an intubated ureteroureterostomy, whereas injuries of the lower third are more often managed with a direct ureterocystoneostomy, with or without a bladder psoas hitch. These techniques are also well suited to injuries diagnosed within 2 weeks of the aetiological trauma. Unfortunately, as stated above, most ureteral injuries may not be recognized or even suspected during surgery as they arise from ligation or fulguration in attempts at haemostasis, or from devascularization while attempting to separate the ureter from malignant tumours.[52] Even small ureteral sections are difficult to notice, as a small urine leakage may easily resemble the normal tissue fluid. As a consequence, more than 80% of iatrogenic injuries to the ureter present postoperatively.[49]

Prognostic factors

In English scientific literature there are only a few publications concerning *prognostic factors* in the management of ureteral injuries diagnosed postoperatively. Contrary to the traditional doctrine of delayed intervention, they report a better outcome for injuries treated in the early postoperative period than for those treated later,[53–56] indicating time of treatment as a valuable prognosticator of treatment outcome. However, in none of these publication has the prognostic value of the time of treatment been statistically analysed. In addition, there is little information regarding the prognostic value of such factors as previous radiotherapy, or site, type and length of the ureteral injury, despite the fact that it is common opinion that all of these may significantly influence the treatment outcome.

The authors have recently analysed the influence of radiotherapy, of site, type and length of the injury, and of time of treatment, on the outcome of 137 ureteral injuries treated in their Division (Tables 2.2 and 2.3) and have statistically evaluated the prognostic significance of these factors.[57]

The length of the lesion was found to be the most important independent prognosticator of treatment outcome (Table 2.4), as failure rate was 60% for injuries longer than 5 cm versus 15% for those shorter than 5 cm ($P < 0.0005$). The unfavourable prognostic value of extensive injury length was probably related to the fact that extensive injuries had to be managed with urinary diversions known to have a high failure rate, or even with primary nephrectomy. Short ureteral injuries, on the contrary, were managed with 'conservative' or reconstructive procedures known to have a low failure rate. In the authors' series the failure rate was 8% (9/106) for those injuries treated with 'conservative' and reconstructive

Aetiology*	No. of patients	Bilateral injury	No. of ureters	Site			Length			Type of injury			
				Upper	Middle	Lower	<2 cm	2–5 cm	>5 cm	Stricture	Avulsion	Fistula	Radiotherapy
O/G	66	19	85	—	3	82	46	30	9	57	—	28	29
U	29	5	34	10	7	17	22	9	3	25	—	9	1
GS	13	—	13	—	6	7	9	3	1	4	—	9	—
O	1	—	1	—	—	1	—	—	1	—	1	—	—
ET	4	—	4	1	2	1	1	2	1	2	—	2	—
Total	113	24	137	11	18	108	78	44	15	88	1	48	30

Table 2.2. Ureteral injuries treated from June 1972 to December 1991
*O/G, obstetric/gynaecological; U, urological; GS, general surgical; O, orthopaedic surgical; ET, external trauma.

Treatment		Complication	
Procedure	No. of ureters	Failure aetiology	No. of ureters
Cystotomy and stenting	9	—	—
Endoscopic stenting	19	—	—
Bladder psoas hitch	41	Stricture of the ureteroneocystostomy	4
Boari flap	2	—	—
Direct ureteroneocystostomy	8	Recurrent UTI*	2
Pyeloplasty	5	—	—
Transureteroureterostomy	3	—	—
Renal pelvis flap	1	—	—
End-to-end ureterostomy	18	Stricture of the ureteroureterostomy	1
		Ureterocutaneous fistula	2
Percutaneous nephrostomy	5	Urinary sepsis (death)	1
Ureterosigmoidostomy	5	Recurrent UTI	2
Ureterocutaneostomy	4	Stricture of the ureterocutaneostomy	1
Uretero-ileocutaneostomy	6	Faecal peritonitis (death)	2
		Urinary sepsis (death)	1
Nephrectomy	11	Nephrectomy	11
Total	137		27

Table 2.3. Treatment and complications of ureteral injuries treated from June 1972 to December 1991
*UTI, urinary tract infection.

procedures, compared with 35% (7/20) for those necessarily treated with diversions.

Previous radiotherapy was also found to be an unfavourable prognostic factor, as the failure rate was 37% for irradiated ureters compared with 15% for those that were not irradiated (P <0.01). Experimental studies[28,29] have proved that the ureter is the most radiation-sensitive abdominal organ and that radiotherapy damages the ureteral vascularization, leading to extensive fibrosis and scarring. Furthermore, surgery in patients with gynaecological malignancies is usually extensive and may already have damaged the ureteral circulation before the administration of radiotherapy. About 50% of the ureteral injuries seen in patients subjected to previous radiotherapy had to be managed with urinary diversions. Thus, the unfavourable prognostic value of radiotherapy, too, may be linked to the high failure rate of these procedures.

Factor		Failure	Success	Total	Significance*
Length	>5 cm	9	6	15	$P < 0.0005$
	<5 cm	18	104	122	
Radiotherapy	Yes	11	19	30	$P < 0.01$
	No	16	91	107	
Treatment	Late	22	58	80	
	Early	5	42	47	$P < 0.05$
	Immediate	—	10	10	
Site	Lower third	22	86	108	NS
	Middle–upper third	5	24	29	
Type of injury	Fistula	7	41	48	
	Stricture	20	68	88	NS
	Avulsion	—	1	1	

Table 2.4. Analysis of prognostic factors for the ureteral injuries treated
*Chi-square test (NS, not significant)

The time of treatment had prognostic significance, as the authors noted that the later the treatment, the higher the failure rate tended to be. In fact, there was no failure among injuries treated immediately, whereas the failure rate was 11% for those treated 'early' and 27% for those treated 'late'. These data confirm that ureteral injuries should be treated as soon as they are diagnosed. The unfavourable prognostic significance of 'late' treatment is generally attributed to fibrosis and scarring of the periureteral tissue or epithelization of a fistulous tract. However, there are grounds for assuming that it may be due, at least in part, to its frequent association with extensive injury length or previous radiotherapy. In the authors' series, injuries diagnosed 'early' were less often extensive or associated with radiotherapy (6%) than those diagnosed 'late' (34%). Consequently, almost all injuries diagnosed 'early' were managed by 'conservative' or reconstructive procedures, whereas one-third of the injuries diagnosed 'late' had to be managed with diversions or even with nephrectomy.

Contrary to expectation, the site and type of injury had no prognostic significance. This observation confirms that there is no significant difference in outcome of the different reconstructive procedures chosen according to the site of the injury.

Treatment

Nowadays, three alternatives are available to the surgeon dealing with a ureteral injury: these are endo-urological treatment, open surgical procedures and even no treatment. The latter applies, for example, to post-radiotherapy partial ureteral strictures in patients with a short life expectancy.

Endo-urological procedures

These have provided new opportunities for repairing ureteral injuries which, until the 1980s, always required open surgery. Andriole and co-workers[58] first reported a 50% success rate in the management of ureteral fistulae with indwelling stents. Dowling and co-workers[3] reported good results in 11 of the 15 ureteral injuries they managed with percutaneous ureteral stenting or with percutaneous nephrostomy drainage alone. In the authors' opinion, percutaneous nephrostomy drainage alone does not lead to restoration of the urinary tract. Experimental studies have proved that proper ureteral regeneration requires urine drainage during the first 4–5 days, to promote epithelialization of the gap, and urine flow during the following 2–3 weeks, to promote regeneration of the muscular layer.[59,60] These goals cannot be achieved by nephrostomy drainage alone.

Chang and co-workers[61] reported successful resolution of 10 of the 12 ureteral fistulae that they treated with percutaneous antegrade ureteral stenting with a double-J catheter. Turner and co-workers[62] have reported good results in nine of 10 ureteral fistulae, following gynaecological surgery, treated with an indwelling double-J stent. Similarly, Toporoff and co-workers[63] have reported good results in five of six late-presenting ureteral injuries secondary to penetrating trauma, which they treated with percutaneous antegrade stenting.

From April 1983 to December 1993, following the trends of modern endo-urology, 34 ureteral injuries were scheduled for endo-urological treatment at the authors' Division (Table 2.5). Attempts to perform ureteral stenting failed in 14 cases (five fistulae and nine strictures). All failures occurred in the case of injuries treated late. Attempts to perform ureteral stenting were successful in 20 lesions, 12 strictures and eight

Aetiology*	No. of patients	Bilateral injury	No. of ureters
O/G	19	4	23
U	5	1	6
GS	4	—	4
ET	1	—	1
Total	29	5	34

Table 2.5. Aetiology of ureteral injuries treated endo-urologically

*O/G, obstetric/gynaecological; U, urological; GS, general surgical; O, orthopaedic surgical; ET, external trauma.

fistulae, 15 of which were treated early and five late. Restoration of a normal urinary tract was achieved in all cases. All patients were followed for 2 years with IVP and ultrasound every 6 months. Significantly, the percentage of ureteral injuries treated by endo-urological methods was 21% (8/38) in the period between April 1983 and December 1989, compared with 63% (12/19) in the period between January 1990 and December 1993.

In the authors' experience, endo-urological treatment has proved to be the ideal therapeutic option for recent injuries less than 2 cm in length.[64] Ureteral fistulae, in which the continuity of the ureteral wall is still partially preserved, have been found to be suitable for endo-urological treatment, as an indwelling double-J stent left in the damaged ureter for 2–3 months promotes recovery with no complications. Injuries due to ligatures or angulations can also benefit from endo-urological treatment if they are recognized and treated early. In fact, within 2–3 weeks of the trauma it is often possible to break the absorbable sutures that caused the ureteral damage, by means of a ureteral stent or a rigid ureterorenoscope, and to complete treatment by placing an indwelling double-J stent. Injuries recognized late are usually complicated by periureteral fibrosis or epithelialization of the fistulous gap. Endo-urological treatment, which can be attempted if the lesion is shorter than 2 cm, generally fails because it is impossible to place the stent. Even in the few cases in which this is possible, long-term results are usually disappointing because of the frequent damage to ureteral vascularization or of tissue retraction due to the scar. It should be observed that such tissue damage can often also bring about the failure of reconstructive surgery. Thus, despite the possibility of failure, frequent only in cases of late treatment of the injury, endo-urological treatment should be considered a safe and effective procedure, well accepted by the patient, that avoids the need for open surgery and its possible complications.

Because endo-urological treatment is simple and relatively non-invasive, work is continuing to extend indications for such treatment to larger injuries. Kramolowsky and co-workers[65] have recently reported successful results in nine (64%) of the 14 ureteral strictures they treated with endoscopic balloon dilatation and subsequent ureteral stenting. Similarly, Netto and co-workers[66] have reported a 57% success rate for ureteral strictures treated with balloon dilatation and subsequent ureteral stenting. Ureteral strictures have also been successfully treated by endoscopic incision and subsequent ureteral stenting[67,68] and, recently, even with indwelling metallic stents. All these techniques are still under investigation and long-term results are not yet available.

Looking to the future, the possibilities of replacing extensive ureteral loss by endoscopic placement of a free urothelial graft mounted on a double-J stent[69] or by urothelial cells seeded on an adsorbable polymer scaffold[70] seem to be of great interest.

Ureteral stenting, however, is not free from problems: migration, encrustation and consequent breakage are well-known complications.[71] Recent reports have outlined the potential of these devices for damaging the uroepithelium,[72] causing urinary tract infections[73] or altering renal pelvic dynamics.[74] Because of the increasing number of double-J stent materials currently available on the market, assurance of their safety should be demanded by clinicians.

In cooperation with a team from Helsinki University (Finland), the authors have recently investigated the safety of various double-J ureteral stents in vivo and in vitro, in terms of alterations of renal pelvic dynamics and renal function, of alterations of the uroepithelium and urine, of bacterial adhesion and of urinary tract infection.

In agreement with previous experimental studies, it was found, in a pig model, that ureteral intubation with a double-J stent results in partial ureteral obstruction and vesico-ureteral reflux, with consequent increase in intrapelvic pressure. Spontaneous adaptation to these changes, consisting of mild ureteral dilatation, and restoration of baseline intrapelvic pressure values, however, occur so fast that renal function is unlikely to be compromised. The study[75] has shown that, perhaps because of their rigidity, pure polyurethane double-J stents may prevent this spontaneous adaptation process and, consequently, may have deleterious effects on renal function.

In vivo in pigs, the authors also found that silicone and hydrogel-coated double-J stents caused less superficial epithelial destruction and inflammatory changes of the uroepithelium than pure polyurethane and 'modified' polyurethane stents, as determined by light microscopy and scanning electron microscopy.[76] Silicone stents, however, were found to be more prone to encrustation than the others, as determined by scanning electron microscopy of the stent surface, and thus to be less suitable than hydrogel-coated stents for long-term ureteral stenting.[76] Cytotoxicity of the stent materials was also studied in vitro on cell cultures.[76] Stents made of 'modified' polyurethane were found to be cytotoxic, whereas stents made of a pure polymer (pure silicone, pure polyurethane) were not, suggesting that plasticizers added to soften the stents are responsible for the toxic effects. Findings in vitro did not correlate with in vivo, probably because of the relatively mild cytotoxicity of the stents and of the effective clearance of the toxic substances in the presence of normal ureteral blood circulation and continuous urinary flow.[76]

In the authors' study in vivo, adhesion of sporadic bacteria occurred on seven of the 23 indwelling double-J stents, and biofilm formation on only two of the 23 indwelling stents, as determined by scanning electron microscopy.[77] Interestingly, only the two renal units intubated with the stents presenting bacterial biofilms yielded positive urine cultures, suggesting that adhesion of sporadic bacteria is of little clinical significance, whereas formation of large bacterial biofilms results in urinary infection. In an assay in vitro, the authors found no statistically significant difference in bacterial adhesion to the various stent materials, showing that the physical or chemical properties of the various test materials do not influence bacterial adhesion. Conversely, there was a statistically significant difference in adhesion among the test bacterial strains, as the two P-fimbriated strains of *Escherichia coli* adhered significantly more than the two without P-fimbriae.[77]

Open surgery

In the case of failure of endo-urological treatment, or of injuries that primarily require open surgery, many factors should be taken into account when choosing the most suitable procedure. First, the patient's general medical condition, life expectancy, and preferences regarding treatment option should be considered. Then, the function and condition of both the affected and the contralateral kidney, as well as the presence of cancer, infection, fibrosis or radiation exposure of the area involved,[51,78] should be taken into account. Obviously, the site and length of the ureteral injury are of major importance in the choice of treatment option.

Once the injury has been fully delineated and the treatment option chosen, several rules for successful surgery should be followed.[51,78] Ureteral mobilization should be minimized to prevent devascularization, but all questionable tissue should be debrided in order to perform anastomoses on well-vascularized ureteral stumps. Care should be taken to create tension-free anastomoses. Too many stitches in the attempt to make the anastomosis watertight should be avoided, as they may compromise the ureteral blood supply and, consequently, the healing process. Finally, omental pedicle sleeves based on the gastro-epiploic vessels increase ureteral blood supply and peristalsis and decrease the risk of fibrosis and urine leakage at the site of the anastomosis.[17]

Short injuries of the distal ureter can be managed using a direct ureteroneocystostomy with an antireflux ureteral reimplantation such as the Politano–Leadbetter procedure, the Paquin procedure or the Lich procedure. The authors do not attempt to repair these injuries with an end-to-end ureterostomy as the distal ureter is often too short, difficult to mobilize and poorly vascularized; they therefore prefer to disregard it.

Whenever the length of the injury precludes the creation of a tension-free anastomosis, a bladder fixation and elongation technique can be performed. The bladder psoas hitch (Fig. 2.1a) has proved to be simpler and safer than the other procedures. Described by Witzel in 1896,[79] it was largely ignored until the enthusiastic reports by Harrow,[80] by Gross and co-workers[81] and, above all, by Turner-Warwick and Worth.[82] In comparison with the Boari flap (Fig. 2.1b), it has the advantages of offering an adequate space for ureteral reimplantation and avoiding the creation of an aperistaltic flap[83] which may undergo ischaemia;[51] in comparison with the Demel flap (Fig. 2.1c) it has the advantage of not involving a long and difficult mobilization of the posterior bladder wall, risking possible neurovascular damage to the ureterovesical junctions. Several authors[84,85] have subsequently supported the efficacy and safety of the bladder psoas hitch and at present it is widely accepted as the procedure of choice for repair of the distal ureter.[51]

Bladder elongation procedures, however, are contraindicated in the case of a neurogenic, tuberculous or irradiated bladder, or in the presence of bladder outlet obstruction.[86]

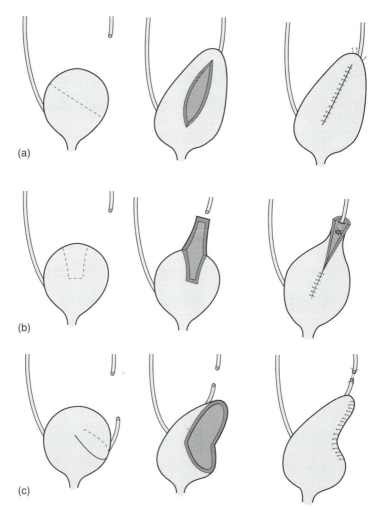

Figure 2.1. Classic bladder elongation procedures: (a) bladder psoas hitch; (b) Boari flap; (c) Demel flap.

Unlike short injuries of the distal ureter, short injuries of the middle ureter can and should be managed with an end-to-end ureterostomy, as the other reconstructive procedures are more difficult to perform and involve a higher risk of complication and failure. In the case of long injuries, on the other hand, the surgeon may choose between several treatment options, such as transureteroureterostomy (TUU), ileal ureter, renal autotransplantation, and combined Boari flap and bladder psoas hitch.

TUU

The results of TUU have varied in different hands. Hendren and Hensle[87] reported good results in 72 (96%) of the 75 patients they treated with TUU. Similarly, Hodges and co-workers[88] reported a 92% success rate for the 100 patients they treated with this procedure; they warned of the dangers of angulating the donor ureter, which should not be placed between the aorta and the inferior mesenteric artery. Conversely, Ehrlich and Skinner[89] and Sandoz and co-workers[90] reported a series of complications and failures following this procedure, mainly due to anastomotic tension, poor blood supply, and injury of the recipient ureter. They also pointed out that unsuccessful TUU may jeopardize the contralateral kidney and consequently lead to renal failure. Moreover, TUU is contraindicated in the case of obstruction of the recipient ureter, retroperitoneal fibrosis or retroperitoneal adenopathy.[17]

Ileal ureter

According to Melnikoff,[91] the first ileal ureter was performed in 1906 by Shoemaker in an 18-year-old girl with urinary tract tuberculosis. The experience gained over the years has shown that the ileum can be interposed in the urinary tract in a variety of ways. The proximal anastomosis may be uretero-ileal, pyelo-ileal, calyco-ileal, or nephro-ileal; the distal anastomosis may be an ileocystostomy or an ileocutaneostomy. Kaufman and co-workers[92] stated that the three most important technical precautions for a successful ileal ureter are that the ileum be used in an isoperistaltic manner, that the bladder be capable of emptying completely, and that the bladder neck be sufficiently patent to allow the passage of mucus produced by the ileum.

The potential drawbacks of this procedure are associated with the inherent properties of the ileum, such as its adsorptive capacity, its mucus production and its tendency to dilate. Resorption of urine by the ileal mucosa may result in hyperchloraemic acidosis and hyperkalaemia. If the renal function is good and the ileal ureter drains well, renal compensation will prevent significant electrolyte abnormalities whereas, if it is impaired, hyperkalaemia may become a major problem. In fact, Boxer and co-workers[93] pointed out that electrolyte problems were unlikely to occur in patients with an ileal ureter, provided that the preoperative creatinine level was below 2.0 mg/100 ml. They reported an 87.5% success rate in patients with preoperative serum creatinine levels lower than 2 mg/100 ml, compared with a 45% success rate in patients with higher serum creatinine levels. Mucus production in combination with bladder outlet obstruction may cause urine retention with consequent excessive electrolyte absorption. The combination of vesico-ileal reflux, always present in these patients, and mucus production, may lead to chronic bacteriuria and, in poorly draining ileal ureters, to recurrent pyelonephritis and renal deterioration.[94] The intestinal segment has a tendency to dilate and thus create high postvoiding residuals, which may lead to acidosis, infection, stone formation and deterioration of the upper tract drainage.[95] Finally, the ileal ureter may undergo neoplastic transformation, albeit after many years.[96]

Shokeir and co-workers[97] have recently suggested the use of a modified valved and tailored ileal ureter. They found this modification to be functionally superior to the standard ileal ureter, as it provided an efficient unidirectional flow of urine from the kidney to the bladder, with less mucus secretion.

Although most experience has been obtained with the ileum, the appendix has also been used successfully for the repair of a damaged right ureter.[98]

Renal autotransplantation

The use of renal autotransplantation for the repair of extensive ureteral injuries has so far been relatively infrequent, with respect to the frequent use of this procedure for the correction of severe renovascular disease. Bodie and co-workers[99] reported a successful outcome in 21 of the 23 patients they treated with renal autotransplantation for ureteral replacement. On the basis of their results, they considered renal autotransplantation a valuable option for the repair of extensive ureteral injuries in young patients without aorto-iliac atherosclerosis, underlying renal disease or retroperitoneal fibrosis. However, retroperitoneal inflammation and scarring, often present in the case of extensive ureteral injuries with massive leakage of urine, may prevent safe donor nephrectomy and renal transplantation.[100]

The combined Boari flap and bladder psoas hitch (Fig. 2.2a)

This was first described by Kelami and co-workers in 1973 in experimental animals.[101] After completing the psoas hitch, a flap was designed with the base (approximately 4 cm in width) at the psoas hitch and the apex (approximately 3 cm in width) directed anteromedially. The flap was then lifted towards the ureteral stump, the ureter anastomosed

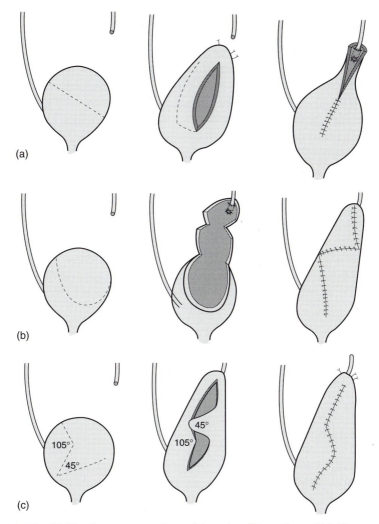

Figure 2.2. New bladder elongation procedures: (a) combined Boari flap and bladder psoas hitch; (b) Passerini–Glazel flap; (c) bladder Z-plasty.

end-to-end or using a submucosal tunnel, and the flap formed into a tube and closed in two layers. Despite the good results reported by Olsson and Norlén,[102] this procedure may have the same drawbacks as the Boari flap, namely stricture of the ureterocystoneostomy, ischaemia of the flap base, and absence of peristalsis in the flap. Moreover, like the other bladder-elongation procedures, it is contraindicated in the case of neurogenic, tuberculous or irradiated bladder, or in the presence of bladder outlet obstruction.

Bladder Z-plasty
Thus, none of the above-mentioned procedures has proved to be

superior to the others. In principle, when planning to replace an extensively injured ureter, the surgeon should always aim to use the bladder, as all other ureteral replacement techniques can involve a number of complications and have a high failure rate. The bladder psoas hitch has proved to be a simple and safe procedure with no significant complications, but it is not suitable for injuries involving the middle third of the ureter. The combined Boari flap and bladder psoas hitch has proved to be suitable for such injuries but may result in a number of complications.

In order to obtain an equally safe but longer bladder elongation than the psoas hitch can provide, the authors studied the mechanisms of bladder elongation in the psoas-hitch procedure on isolated pig bladders.[103] They found that bladder elongation was 75% due to bladder stretching and 25% due to the bladder incision, and that it was impossible to stretch the bladder further, whereas it would be possible to realize a more advantageous bladder incision. Considering the good results obtained in plastic and orthopaedic surgery by the Z-plasties, different Z-shaped bladder incisions were attempted until the most advantageous was found.[103] In a subsequent study,[104] the authors performed this bladder Z-plasty in sheep to evaluate its efficacy and safety in vivo. After preoperative cystography, surgery was carried out under subarachnoid lumbosacral anaesthesia.[105] Five sheep underwent the psoas-hitch procedure. Ureteral reimplantation was not performed, to avoid confounding factors. Bladder Z-plasty was carried out in a further six sheep as follows (Fig. 2.2c): (a) the upper line of the 'Z' was incised on the bladder dome, half on the anterior and half on the posterior wall, perpendicular to the required elongation axis; (b) the middle line was incised on the anterior wall up the lower margin, creating an angle of approximately 105 degrees with the upper line; (c) the lower line was incised along the entire anterior wall, creating an angle of approximately 45 degrees with the middle line. The centre of the upper line was lifted towards the injured ureter and the position of the middle and inferior bladder flaps was inverted to give the bladder a tubular shape. Finally, the bladder was closed with continuous 2/0 chromic catgut and fixed to the psoas tendon with a few 0 Dexon stitches.

As previously stated, in the first three sheep with the Z-plasty, ureteral reimplantation was not performed, so that the bladder elongation technique could be evaluated without having to take any other factors into consideration. After having ascertained the simplicity of the bladder elongation with Z-plasty in these first three sheep, the other three were subjected to ureteral reimplantation also. Retrograde cystograms, performed 3 weeks after the operation, showed that the Z-plasty provided a mean of 5.8 cm greater bladder elongation than the psoas-hitch procedure.

Analysing the mechanisms of bladder elongation in the Z-plasty procedure, it can be seen that, basically, it results from the creation of three large flaps. The upper flap, as in the Demel technique, can be turned up towards the damaged ureter but its high position avoids extensive dissection of the posterior bladder wall, while its shape avoids the risk of ischaemia or necrosis of the flap base. Moreover, when it is sutured together with the previously inverted middle and inferior flaps, the bladder takes on a tubular shape, becoming a dynamic 'reservoir' that, by contracting, eliminates the non-peristaltic tubularized flap, which is a characteristic drawback of the Boari procedure.[83] The width of the upper flap allows a safe antireflux ureteroneocystostomy, while the shape of the middle and inferior flaps ensures good vascularization and the absence of stenosis of their base. Finally, as in the bladder psoas-hitch procedure, the entire tubular bladder can be lifted towards the damaged ureter and fixed to the psoas tendon, obtaining an equally safe but greater elongation.

On the basis of the good results obtained in sheep, the authors recently performed a bladder Z-plasty in a 60-year-old woman who had a right ureterocutaneostomy, performed in a country hospital to manage an extensive injury of the right ureter due to ureteroscopy (Fig. 2.3). The elongated bladder reached almost to the lower pole of the kidney (Fig. 2.4). One year after surgery the patient is doing well. This experience in a human confirms the efficacy of the technique for the repair of extensive ureteral injuries.

Although the management of extensive injuries has become easier, the management of bilateral injuries can still be problematic. In the authors' opinion, bilateral injuries can be subdivided into 'easy' and 'complicated'. The former are those shorter than 5 cm, diagnosed early, in patients who have not undergone radiotherapy; they can be successfully treated like unilateral injuries, with endo-urological procedures or with bilateral bladder elongation procedures. The latter, conversely, are those longer than 5 cm, diagnosed late and seen in patients who have undergone radiotherapy; they usually require the interposition of intestinal segments, with their related complications. In such high-risk patients, life expectancy is probably the main criterion on which to base the choice of treatment. In severe cases, nothing more ambitious than a percutaneous nephrostomy or, at most, a subcutaneous nephrovesical diversion, should be attempted.[106]

Conclusions

In conclusion, it is the authors' opinion that, whereas injuries recognized intra-operatively can be treated by the surgeon who generated them, provided that he has some experience in this matter, injuries recognized postoperatively or late may be very complicated and require a skilled urologist with extensive experience.

To sum up, over the last 22 years, the authors have learned the following rules of thumb in the management of ureteral injuries:

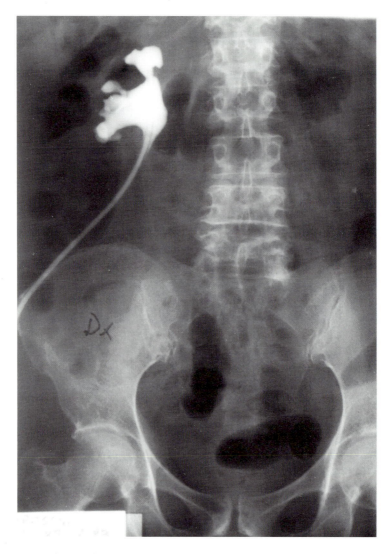

Figure 2.3. Intubated right ureterocutaneostomy performed to manage an extensive injury to the right ureter due to ureteroscopy.

1. *Do not attempt to treat an injury by nephrostomy drainage alone.* Only a few injuries will resolve spontaneously after readsorption of the suture material, and nephrostomy drainage is not without complications.
2. In injuries diagnosed in the early postoperative period, *do not wait until stabilization of the injury but treat as soon as possible.* The traditional doctrine of delayed intervention, which is appropriate for postpartum vesicovaginal fistulae, has long been applied to all ureteral injuries in order to avoid tissue inflammation and infection. The authors' data, and

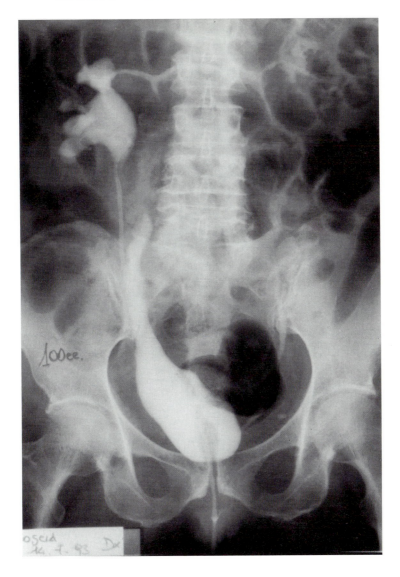

Figure 2.4. Postoperative retrograde cystography. The elongated bladder reaches almost to the lower pole of the kidney.

those of other authors, support early intervention to avoid the development of peri-ureteral fibrosis, which would render surgery more difficult and prone to failure.

3. *Always try to use the bladder for replacement of the damaged pelvic ureter.* The distal ureter can be difficult to mobilize and is often short and poorly vascularized; the authors prefer to disregard it. Other procedures, such as interposition of bowel segments, kidney autotransplantation and transureteroureterostomy, involve a high risk of complication and failure.

35

4. *The bladder should be elongated and fixed.* Elongation provides the possibility of reaching a healthy ureteral stump, while fixation to the psoas tendon is of major importance to stabilize the elongation and, above all, the ureterovesical anastomosis. For these reasons, the authors perform direct ureteroneocystostomies only in cases of very distal lesions. In their experience, the bladder psoas hitch has proved to be a safe and effective procedure. If necessary, greater elongation can be achieved by using flaps, such as the combined Boari flap and bladder psoas hitch, or the extended Boari flap[107] with lateral and medial incisions (Fig. 2.2b) or the authors' bladder Z-plasty, described here.

References

1. Wertheim F. Zer frage der radikaloperation bei uteruskrebs. Arch Gynecol 1900; 61: 627–631

2. Schmitz H. The classification of uterine carcinoma for the efficacy of radiation therapy. Am J Roentgenol 1920; 7: 383–390

3. Dowling R A, Corriere J N, Sandler C M. Iatrogenic ureteral injury. J Urol 1986; 135: 912–915

4. Solomons E, Levin E J, Bauman J, Baron J. A pyelographic study of ureteral injuries sustained during hysterectomy for benign conditions. Surg Gynecol Obstet 1960; 111: 41–48

5. Mann W J, Arato M, Patsner B, Stone M L. Ureteral injuries in an obstetrics and gynecology training program: etiology and management. Obstet Gynecol 1988; 72: 82–85

6. Daly J W, Higgins K A. Injury to the ureter during gynecologic surgical procedures. Surg Gynecol Obstet 1988; 167: 19–22

7. Tarkington M A, Dejter S W, Bresette J F. Early surgical management of extensive gynecologic ureteral injuries. Surg Gynecol Obstet 1991; 173: 17–21

8. Eisenkop S M, Richman P, Platt L D, Paul R H. Urinary tract injury during cesarean section. Obstet Gynecol 1982; 60: 591–596

9. St Martin E C, Trichel B E, Campbell J H, Locke C H. Ureteral injuries in gynecologic surgery. J Urol 1953; 70: 51–57

10. Riss P, Koelbl H, Neunteufel W, Janisch H. Wertheim radical hysterectomy 1921–1986: changes in urological complications. Arch Gynecol Obstet 1988; 241: 249–253

11. Gangi M P, Agee R E, Spence C R. Surgical injury to the ureter. Urology 1976; 8: 22–27

12. Boyd M E. Care of the ureter in pelvic surgery. Can J Surg 1987; 30: 234–236

13. Neuman M, Eidelman A, Langer R et al. Iatrogenic injuries to the ureter during gynecologic and obstetric operations. Surg Gynecol Obstet 1991; 173: 268–272

14. Symmonds R E. Ureteral injuries associated with gynecologic surgery: prevention and management. Clin Obstet Gynecol 1976; 19: 623–644

15. Hughes E S R, McDermott F T, Polglase A L, Johnson W R. Ureteral damage in surgery for cancer of the large bowel. Dis Colon Rectum 1984; 27: 293–295

16. Andersson Å, Bergdahl L. Urologic complications following abdomino-perineal resection of the rectum. Arch Surg 1976; 111: 969–971

17. Zinman L M, Libertino J A, Roth R A. Management of operative ureteral injury. Urology 1978; 12: 290–303

18. Higgins C C. Ureteral injuries during surgery. JAMA 1967; 199: 118–124

19. Spence H M, Boone T. Surgical injuries to the ureter. JAMA 1961; 176: 1070–1076

20. Nicely E P. Injuries of the ureter following pelvic surgery. J Urol 1950; 64: 283–288

21. Heard G, Hinde G. Hydronephrosis complicating aortic reconstruction. Br J Surg 1975; 62: 344–347

22. Goldenberg S L, Gordon P B, Cooperberg P L, McLoughlin M G. Early hydronephrosis following aortic bifurcation graft surgery: a prospective study. J Urol 1988; 140: 1367–1369

23. Blasco F J, Saladie J M. Ureteral obstruction and ureteral fistulas after aortofemoral or aortoiliac bypass surgery. J Urol 1991; 145: 237–242

24. Smith A D. Management of iatrogenic ureteral strictures after urological procedures. J Urol 1988; 140: 1372–1374
25. Rhamy R, Stander R. Pyelographic analysis of radiation therapy in carcinoma of the cervix. Am J Roentgenol 1962; 87: 41–43
26. Shingleton H, Fowler W C, Pepper F D, Palumbo L. Ureteral strictures following therapy for carcinoma of the cervix. Cancer 1969; 24: 77–83
27. Weed J. Treatment of stage I and stage II carcinoma of the cervix: the results of combined irradiation and surgical treatment. Pacific Med Surg 1967; 75: 319–326
28. Gillette S L, Gillette E L, Powers B E et al. Ureteral injuries following experimental intraoperative radiation. Int J Radiat Oncol Biol Phys 1989; 17: 791–798
29. Hoekstra H J, Mehta D M, Oosterhuis J W et al. The short and long term effect of single high-dose intraoperative electron beam irradiation on retroperitoneal structures: an experimental study in dogs. Eur J Surg Oncol 1990; 16: 240–247
30. Brady L W, Farber S H. Ureteral injury as a consequence of radiation therapy. In: Bergman H (ed) The ureter. New York: Springer-Verlag, 1981: 421–426
31. Graham J B, Abad R S. Ureteral obstruction due to radiation. Am J Obstet Gynecol 1967; 99: 409–412
32. Huffman J L. Ureteroscopic injuries to the upper urinary tract. Urol Clin North Am 1989; 16: 249–254
33. Kramolowsky E V. Ureteral perforation during ureterorenoscopy: treatment and management. J Urol 1987; 138: 36–38
34. Egawa S, Shiokawa H, Uchida T et al. Delayed presentation of ureteral injury following arthrodesis of the hip joint. Br J Urol 1994; 73: 212–213
35. Carrieri G, Callea A, Gala F et al. Avulsione dell'uretere pelvico in corso di artroprotesi dell'anca. Atti Soc Urol It Centro Mer Isole 1986; 22: 269–273
36. Stengel J N, Felderman E S, Zamora D. Ureteral injury. Complication of laparoscopic sterilization. Urology 1974; 4: 341–344
37. Steckel J, Badillo F, Waldbaum R S. Uretero-fallopian tube fistula secondary to laparoscopic fulguration of pelvic endometriosis. J Urol 1993; 149: 1128–1129
38. Woodland M B. Ureter injury during laparoscopic-assisted vaginal hysterectomy with the endoscopic linear stapler. Am J Obstet Gynecol 1992; 167: 756–757
39. Dogra P M, Jadeja N A. Urosepsis and ureteral strictures following extracorporeal shock wave lithotripsy. Eur Urol 1994; 52: 109–112
40. Jones W R, Haines C J, Matthews C D, Kirby C A. Traumatic ureteral obstruction secondary to oocyte recovery for in vitro fertilization: a case report. J In Vitro Fert Embryo Transf 1989; 6: 185–187
41. Trigaux J P, Decoene B, van Beers B. Focal necrosis of the ureter following CT-guided chemical sympathectomy. Cardiovasc Intervent Radiol 1992; 15: 180–182
42. Walk W L, Foret J D. The problem of vesico-vaginal and uretero-vaginal fistulas. Med Clin North Am 1959; 43: 1765–1769
43. Remington J H. Prevention of ureteral injury in surgery of the pelvic colon. Dis Colon Rectum 1959; 2: 340–349
44. Leff E I, Groff W, Rubin R J et al. Use of ureteral catheters in colonic and rectal surgery. Dis Colon Rectum 1982; 25: 457–460
45. Selvaggi F P, Battaglia M, Traficante A et al. Obstetric and gynecological lesions of the ureter: experience with 88 injuries. Int Urogynecol J 1991; 2: 81–84
46. Sheikh F A, Khubchandani I T. Prophylactic ureteral catheters in colon surgery—how safe are they? Report of three cases. Dis Colon Rectum 1990; 33: 508–510
47. Phipps J H, Tyrrell N J. Transilluminating ureteral stents for preventing operative ureteral damage. Br J Obstet Gynaecol 1992; 99: 81
48. Hoch W H, Kursh E D, Persky L. Early aggressive management of intraoperative ureteral injuries. J Urol 1975; 114: 530–532
49. Witters S, Cornelissen M, Vereecken R. Iatrogenic ureteral injury: aggressive or conservative treatment. Am J Obstet Gynecol 1986; 155: 582–584
50. McAninch J W. Injuries to the genitourinary tract. In: Tanagho E A, McAninch J W (eds) Smith's General urology. Norwalk, Ct: Appleton and Lange, 1988: 302–318
51. Lezin M A, Stoller M L. Surgical ureteral injuries. Urology 1991; 38: 497–506

52. Cruikshank S H. Avoiding ureteral injury during total vaginal hysterectomy. South Med J 1985; 78: 1447–1450
53. Badenoch D F, Tiptaft R C, Thakar D R et al. Early repair of accidental injury to the ureter or bladder following gynaecological surgery. Br J Urol 1987; 59: 516–518
54. Beland G. Early treatment of ureteral injuries found after gynecological surgery. J Urol 1977; 118: 25–27
55. Blandy J P, Badenoch D F, Fowler C G et al. Early repair of iatrogenic injury to the ureter or bladder after gynecological surgery. J Urol 1991; 146: 761–765
56. Flynn J T, Tiptaft R C, Woodhouse C R J et al. Early and aggressive repair of iatrogenic ureteral injuries. Br J Urol 1979; 51: 454–457
57. Cormio L, Ruutu M, Selvaggi F P. Prognostic factors in the management of ureteral injuries. Ann Chir Gynaecol 1994; 83: 41–44
58. Andriole G L, Bettmann M A, Garnick M B, Richie J P. Indwelling double-J ureteral stents for temporary and permanent urinary drainage: experience with 87 patients. J Urol 1984; 131: 239–241
59. Oppenheimer R, Hinman F Jr. The effect of urinary flow upon ureteral regeneration in the absence of splint. Surg Gynecol Obstet 1956; 103: 416–422
60. Hinman F Jr, Oppenheimner R O F. Ureteral regeneration. VI. Delayed urinary flow in the healing of unsplinted ureteral defects. J Urol 1957; 78: 138–144
61. Chang R, Marshall F F, Mitchell S. Percutaneous management of benign ureteral strictures and fistulas. J Urol 1987; 137: 1126–1131
62. Turner W H, Cranston D W, Davies A H et al. Double-J stents in the treatment of gynaecological injury to the ureter. J R Soc Med 1990; 83: 623–624
63. Toporoff B, Sclafani S, Scalea T et al. Percutaneous antegrade ureteral stenting as an adjunct for treatment of complicated ureteral injuries. J Trauma 1992; 32: 534–538
64. Cormio L, Battaglia M, Traficante A, Selvaggi F P. Endourological treatment of ureteral injuries. Br J Urol 1993; 72: 165–168
65. Kramolowsky E V, Tucker R D, Nelson C M K. Management of benign ureteral strictures: open surgical repair or endoscopic dilation? J Urol 1989; 141: 285–286
66. Netto N R Jr, Ferreira U, Lemos G C, Claro J F A. Endourological management of ureteral strictures. J Urol 1990; 144: 631–634
67. Schneider A W, Busch R, Otto U, Klosterhalfen H. Endourological management of 41 stenoses in the upper urinary tract using the cold knife technique. J Urol 1989; 141: 208A (abstr 155)
68. Franco I, Eshghi M, Schwalb D, Addonizio J C. Cold knife endoureterotomy of 28 ureteral strictures. J Urol 1989; 141: 208A (abstr 158)
69. Urban D A, Kerbl K, Clayman R V, McDougall E. Endo-ureteroplasty with a free urothelial graft. J Urol 1994; 152: 910–915
70. Atala A, Vacanti J P, Peters C A et al. Formation of urothelial structures in vivo from dissociated cells attached to biodegradable polymer scaffolds in vitro. J Urol 1992; 148: 658–662
71. Saltzman B. Ureteral stents. Indications, variations and complications. Urol Clin North Am 1988; 15: 481–491
72. Marx M, Bettmann M A, Bridge S et al. The effects of various indwelling ureteral catheter materials on the normal canine ureter. J Urol 1988; 139: 180–185
73. Reid G, Denstedt J D, Kang Y S et al. Microbial adhesion and biofilm formation on ureteral stents in vitro and in vivo. J Urol 1992; 148: 1592–1594
74. Payne S R, Ramsay J W A. The effects of double J stents on renal pelvic dynamics in the pig. J Urol 1988; 140: 637–641
75. Cormio L, Koivusalo A, Mäkisalo H et al. The effects of various indwelling JJ stents on renal pelvic pressure and renal parenchymal thickness in the pig. Br J Urol 1994; 74: 440–443
76. Cormio L, Talja M, Koivusalo A et al. Biocompatibility of various indwelling double-J stents. J Urol 1995; 153: 494–496
77. Cormio L, Vuopio-Varkila J, Siitonen A et al. Bacterial adhesion and biofilm formation on various double-J stents in vivo and in vitro. Scand J Urol Nephrol 1995; in press
78. Selvaggi F P, Traficante A, Battaglia M et al. Early treatment of ureteral injuries. Proc 20th Congr SIU, Wien 1985, 135–136

79. Witzel O. Extraperitoneale ureterocystostomie mit schrägkanalbildung. Zentralbl Gynakol 1896; 20: 189–193
80. Harrow B R. A neglected maneuver for ureterovesical reimplantation following injury at gynecologic operations. J Urol 1968; 100: 280–284
81. Gross M, Peng B, Waterhouse K. Use of the mobilized bladder to replace the pelvic ureter. J Urol 1969; 101: 40–44
82. Turner-Warwick R, Worth P H L. The psoas bladder-hitch procedure for the replacement of the lower third of the ureter. Br J Urol 1969; 41: 701–709
83. Weinberg S R, Rosemberg J W. Injuries of the ureter. In: Bergman H (ed) The ureter. New York: Springer-Verlag, 1981; 427–448
84. Kishev S V. Psoas-bladder hitch procedure: our experience with the injured ureter in men. J Urol 1975; 113: 772–776
85. Ehrlich R M, Melman A, Skinner D G. The use of vesico-psoas hitch in urologic surgery. J Urol 1978; 119: 322–325
86. Boxer R J, Johnson S F, Ehrlich R M. Ureteral substitution. Urology 1978; 12: 269–271
87. Hendren W H, Hensle T W. Transureteroureterostomy: experience with 75 cases. J Urol 1980; 123: 826–833
88. Hodges C V, Barry J M, Fuchs E F et al. Transureteroureterostomy: 25-year experience with 100 patients. J Urol 1980; 123: 834–838
89. Ehrlich R M, Skinner D G. Complications of transureteroureterostomy. J Urol 1975; 113: 467–473
90. Sandoz I L, Paull D P, MacFarlane C A. Complications with transureteroureterostomy. J Urol 1977; 117: 39–42
91. Melnikoff A E. Sur le replacement de l'uretère par une anse isolée de l'intestin grêle. Rev Clin Urol 1912; 1: 601–605
92. Kaufman J J, Ehrlich R M, Boxer R J. Ureteral replacements. In: Bergman H (ed) The ureter. New York: Springer-Verlag, 1981; 655–668
93. Boxer R J, Fritzsche P, Skinner D G et al. Replacement of the ureter by small intestine: clinical application and results of the ileal ureter in 89 patients. J Urol 1979; 121: 728–731
94. Prout G R Jr, Stuart W T, Witus W S. Utilization of ileal segments to substitute for extensive ureteral loss. J Urol 1963; 90: 541–551
95. Tanagho E A. A case against incorporation of bowel segments into the closed urinary system. J Urol 1975; 113: 796–802
96. Filmer R B, Spencer J R. Malignancies in bladder augmentations and intestinal conduits. J Urol 1990; 143: 671–678
97. Shokeir A A, Gaballah M A, Ashamallah A A, Ghoneim M A. Optimization of replacement of the ureter by ileum. J Urol 1991; 146: 306–310
98. Komatz Y, Itoh H. A case of ureteral injury repaired with appendix. J Urol 1990; 144: 132–133
99. Bodie B, Novick A C, Rose M, Straffon R A. Long-term results of renal autotransplantation for ureteral replacement. J Urol 1986; 136: 1187–1189
100. Stewart B H. Autotransplantation for extensive ureteral disease. In: Bergman H (ed) The ureter. New York: Springer-Verlag, 1981; 449–459
101. Kelami A, Fiedler U, Schmidt V et al. Replacement of the ureter using the urinary bladder. Urol Res 1973; 1: 161–165
102. Olsson C A, Norlén L J. Combined Boari bladder flap–psoas bladder hitch procedure in ureteral replacement. Scand J Urol Nephrol 1986; 20: 279–284
103. Selvaggi F P, Traficante A, Battaglia M et al. Z-plasty procedure to elongate bladder: an experimental model. Eur Urol 1990; 18(suppl. 1): 310
104. Cormio L, Crovace A, Lacalandra G et al. Bladder Z-plasty for the repair of ureteral injuries. Experimental study in sheep. Br J Urol 1993; 71: 667–671
105. Crovace A, Di Bello A, Boscia D, Mastronardi M. Rachianestesia lombosacrale negli ovini. SUMMA 1989; 6: 49–51
106. Cormio L, Ruutu M, Traficante A et al. Management of bilateral ureteral injuries after gynaecological and obstetric procedures. Int Urol Nephrol 1993; 25: 551–555
107. Passerini-Glazel G, Meneghini A, Aragona F et al. Technical options in complex ureteral lesions: ureter sparing surgery. Eur Urol 1994; 25: 273–280

Complications of endoscopic urological surgery and laparoscopic surgery

3

K. Bandhauer

Introduction

Discussion of the major potential complications of endoscopic urological surgery and laparoscopy should cover almost all current urological procedures done by scopes either inside the urinary tract, in the peritoneal cavity or in the retroperitoneal space. Because this subject is so extensive, only those procedures that are already an integral part of urological practice are discussed here; these include diagnostic and therapeutic ureteroscopy and laparoscopic pelvic lymph node dissection.

Ureteroscopy

Ureteroscopic procedures for diagnostic and therapeutic purposes, especially for the removal of ureteral calculi, were introduced into the armamentarium of urology at almost the same time as percutaneous stone removal (litholapaxy) and extracorporeal shock-wave lithotripsy (ESWL). Small-calibre (7.2–9.5 Ch) rod lens ureteroscopes are now in use and advanced fibre-optic technology has provided a new generation of flexible and semi-rigid fibre-optic ureteroscopes. Although there is little debate concerning the appropriate selection of ureteroscopic instrumentation, the devices for intra-ureteral stone fragmentation provide significantly more controversy. Ultrasonic, electrohydraulic and laser lithotripsy have been used with increasing success and a lower complication rate. Since 1990 the Swiss lithoclast has been improved technically to provide successful fragmentation of more than 90% of urinary stones. In the author's own experience, a success rate of more than 90% can be expected with the Swiss lithoclast for fragmentation of ureteral stones.[1,2]

For the management of ureteral calculi and success with regard to stone-free rates location of the calculi is important. For treatment of upper ureteral calculi, ESWL in situ is the procedure of choice, with or without auxiliary measures such as pushback of the stone into the renal pelvis or double-J stents. For stones in mid-ureter, ESWL is also the therapy of choice, although ureteroscopy offers excellent stone-free rates but is more invasive. With the last generation of lithotriptors with integrated X-ray equipment, it has become easier to focus on stones in the middle part of the ureter. For distal ureteral calculi, ESWL is certainly an excellent option but

40

without any doubt the immediate stone-free rate is higher and approaching 100% with ureteroscopy.[3,4]

Complications of ureteroscopy and other endoscopic procedures

Complications of ureteroscopic stone manipulation have varied from minor complications such as haematuria, urinary infection and ureteral colic to major complications such as extended mucosal laceration (especially at the ureteral ostium and at the crossing of ureter and iliac vessels) and perforation of the ureter (mostly at the site of the ureteral stone).[5–10]

Whereas minor complications can be treated by observation only, in most cases, and need no endoscopic or surgical intervention, the management of the major local complications depends primarily on the extent of the lesion, on its location, and on whether the stone has been removed.

Mucosal lacerations

Mucosal lacerations, mostly following stone extraction by forceps or baskets with trapping of the ureteral wall (immediately suspected when significant amounts of blood-stained urine spurt out of the manipulated ureter) can be treated by a double-J stent for 3–5 days.

Perforations

Perforation of the ureter during ureteroscopy occurs in approximately 5–10% of procedures. Two segments of the ureter are particularly at risk of perforation, either during insertion of the guidewire or by the ureteroscope. These are: (a) the distal segment up to about 5 cm from the bladder wall, where the ureter might adhere following previous manipulations causing a periureteral reaction, or where stones may become lodged, and (b) the segment where the ureter crosses the iliac vessels.

The major risk of perforation lies in the extravasation of irrigation fluid and urine and long-term formation of peri-ureteral fibrosis, with occlusion of the ureteral lumen.[8]

Minor perforations, when noted during advancement of the ureteroscope, can be bridged with a double-J stent after removal of the stone. No other treatment is necessary in most cases and when the stent is removed, after 10–12 days, there is usually no extravasation visible on intravenous pyelography.

Major perforations usually do not allow the insertion of a double-J stent and it is dangerous to attempt this by force. The therapy of choice is a percutaneous nephrostomy for at least 5–6 days. When antegrade ureterography then shows no extravasation and/or free drainage, the nephrostomy drain can be clamped, and removed after several hours when no pain or fever have occurred. If extravasation is still visible after more than 6 days the insertion of a double-J stent is advisable, leaving the nephrostomy tube in place. After about 2 weeks the stent can be removed and the complete closure of the perforation can be monitored by antegrade ureterography.

Severe ureteral injuries may occur as a result of perforation of the ureteral wall when the laceration is missed and forcible manipulation is continued to remove the stone.[4,5,8,9]

Avulsion

The inappropriate use of stone-baskets and the extraction of large stones by forceps can lead to complete avulsion of the ureter. When an immediate repair is not indicated because of general or local contraindications, a percutaneous nephrostomy should be placed to salvage renal function until reconstructive surgery is possible.

Stricture

Stricture formation associated with perforation is a very rare event when the perforation is managed correctly. Although most authors have not observed any stricture after ureterosopy, Kramolovsky reported a 5% stricture rate.[11] Strictures occur mostly in the first 6 weeks after ureteroscopy and should be treated as early as possible. A balloon dilatation with a success rate of about 50–60% or cutting techniques with knives or endoscopic scissors, with success rates from 60 to 80%, are indicated, depending on the location of the stricture.[4,9]

Obliteration

Complete obliteration of the ureter after ureteroscopic manipulation is a rare complication and occurs when a severe laceration of the ureteral wall is missed or after complete avulsion of the ureter. In the literature only case reports are published, no precise rates of obliteration being reported. It is probable that some cases of complete obliteration are grouped with those cases of strictures needing surgery. Although some strictures of the ureter, as already mentioned, can be managed by balloon dilatation or knife incision, complete obliteration always needs surgical intervention, depending on where the occlusion is located. In the distal part of the ureter, ureterocystoneostomy is the treatment of choice, whereas in the middle or upper ureter the obliterated part can be resected and an end-to-end anastomosis can be performed.

Ureteral dilatation

There is some discussion about the necessity for, and the mode of, ureteral dilatation before ureteroscopy.[12] Schwalb et al.[13] investigated the gross and microscopic effects of different modes of ureteral dilatation for ureteroscopy in minipigs. Two weeks after mechanical dilatation with bougie, Teflon or balloon and ureterorenoscopy (URS), three of six ureters were found to be obstructed, as assessed radiographically, whereas hydraulically dilated ureters were not obstructed. Although by 6 weeks the radiographic evidence of obstruction had resolved, the mechanically dilated ureters showed extensive scarring with muscle loss, whereas no scarring was seen in those ureters dilated hydraulically. These results seem of interest and correspond to the author's clinical observation of a higher risk of scar formation after mechanical dilatation of the distal ureter. Hydraulic dilatation for URS is less dangerous than mechanical manipulation. In the author's institution hydraulic dilatation by Ureteromat is the preferred procedure, with no complications so far.

Elevated renal pelvic pressure (> 200 cmH$_2$O or 150 mmHg) caused flattening of the calyceal urothelium and submucosal oedema, with, 4–6 weeks later, a higher incidence of columnar metaplasia, subepithelial nests and pericalyceal vasculitis. Renal tubules subjected to high irrigant pressure demonstrated marked vacuolization and degeneration with focal scarring. Irrigation pressure during URS should therefore be kept as low as possible (< 120 cmH$_2$O or 90 mmHg).[13]

Septicaemia

Another major complication of ureteroscopy, irrespective of the indication (stone extraction, endoscopic treatment of ureteral tumours, etc.) is severe urinary tract infection leading to septicaemia. Immediate urinary drainage by percutaneous nephrostomy and adjusted parenteral antibiotic therapy will manage this otherwise fatal complication successfully.

Relative lack of complications

Ureteroscopic therapy of ureteral stones is, after a learning curve, a fairly safe procedure with only a few serious complications. Even bilateral same-session ureteroscopy can be performed, therefore, with a low complication rate. Camilleri et al.[14] reported bilateral same-session ureteroscopy in 13 patients without major short-term or long-term complications. Because of the decreasing complication rate of ureteroscopy, due both to the increased experience of the urologist and to smaller instruments, URS can be considered even as an outpatient procedure in patients without pre-existing risk factors. Wills and Burns,[15] reporting on 134 patients treated as outpatients, achieved a rehospitalization rate of only 3%. In spite of this improvement in the technique of ureteroscopy for stone removal, the experienced endoscopist should bear in mind the possibility of complications that will require specific appropriate treatment.

Stone migration

Stone migration during ureteroscopic stone manipulation can occur in all parts of the ureter, most frequently in the upper third. When the stone is dislocated into the renal pelvis it is easier to insert a double-J catheter and to treat the stone by ESWL than to attempt time-consuming procedures to locate and extract the stone by URS.

ESWL

Although ureteroscopy provides a successful rate of stone removal—close to 100%—with a low incidence of major complications, it is nevertheless an invasive procedure with some risk factors. Conversely, ESWL offers a minimally invasive and very effective option for treatment of calculi all across the ureter. ESWL requires less than half the operating time and is safer than ureteroscopy. Although the stone-free rate is somewhat lower with ESWL, reported as between 85 and 100%, and requires sometimes two or more sessions, ESWL is the first treatment option for ureteral calculi independent of the stone location. Ureteroscopy should be reserved for those patients who either fail therapy with ESWL in situ or need acute removal of the stone because of complete ureteral obstruction with the onset of symptoms of septicaemia.

Percutaneous endopyelotomy

Percutaneous endopyelotomy to treat stenoses at the ureteral pelvic junction was introduced as a clinically useful method by different authors.[16-22] The results of endopyelotomy are most encouraging and the success rate is as high as 85–90%. The complication rate after a learning curve is low and corresponds to the complications of ureteroscopy. Because the complication rate after endoscopic pyelotomy is higher in the treatment of primary stenoses, the novice should initially deal with secondary stenoses that result after unsuccessful open pyeloplasties.

Urothelial tumours

Endourological management of upper tract urothelial tumours, either by ureteroscopy or by the percutaneous approach, is recommended as a conservative parenchyma-sparing method for low-grade non-invasive lesions, especially for those patients with a single kidney, renal insufficiency or bilateral tumours.[23]

Several complications may occur with ureteroscopic management of upper urinary tract tumours, including perforations and strictures, which are rarely reported. Electrocoagulation or laser photocoagulation may be used to ablate the tumours, and supplementary therapy with postoperative instillations of BCG and mitomycin C is under discussion. Increasing pressure due to the irrigation necessary for visualization may increase the renal pelvic pressure, resulting in pyelovenous lymphatic backflow.

One case has been reported of renal pelvic transitional cell carcinoma that may have migrated to the submucosal venous and lymphatic spaces during flexible ureterorenoscopy.[24]

No long-term results are available at present and the majority of patients with upper tract urothelial tumours are still best treated by nephroureterectomy.

Balloon catheter dilatation

Balloon catheter dilatation is recommended for ureteral strictures of various origins, even for strictures that have developed after renal transplantation.[25] If necessary, a balloon catheter dilatation can be followed by placement of a ureteral stent. About 50% of ureteral strictures can successfully be dilated for insertion of a stent. Strictures of the intramural part of the ureter or developing at the ureteroneostomy site respond favourably more often than do strictures in other locations—at least temporarily. Upper urinary tract obstructions that cannot be dilated by the retrograde route can be treated with metallic self-expandable stents.[26,27] The use of self-expandable ureteral stents percutaneously implanted with or without a double-J stent alleviates upper urinary tract obstruction and avoids external urinary drainage. The use of this stent should be reserved for palliative therapy in malignant diseases of the small part of the bony pelvis.

The most frequent complications of ureteral stents are recurrent strictures by scar formation, imperfect drainage, migration of the stent and unpredictable biocompatibility. All patients with intraluminal stents in the urinary tract therefore require close clinical sonographic and radiological monitoring and, where severe complications arise, the stent should be removed immediately.

Conclusions

In conclusion, ureteroscopy and other endoscopic procedures within the upper urinary tract, despite several complications, constitute an important advance in the diagnosis and treatment of different diseases. With increasing experience the frequency of complications should be reduced to a minimum. Nevertheless, every urologist performing endoureteral procedures should be aware that complications may occur and that their early detection and appropriate treatment is crucial for success.

Complications of laparoscopic pelvic lymph node dissection

Urologists are using operative laparoscopy more frequently to diagnose and treat different diseases that traditionally have been approached by open surgery.[28,29] Capelouto and Kavoussi[30] have given an excellent summary of the problems, pitfalls and complications of laparoscopic surgery. In this chapter it is not possible to review all the major complications of laparo-scopic surgery, and the chapter is therefore restricted to the problems and complications of pelvic laparoscopy, and to those of laparoscopic pelvic lymph node dissection in particular. Since 1991, when Schüssler et al.[31] described laparoscopic pelvic lymph node dissection, this method has gained increasing importance for staging prostate and bladder cancer.[32–34]

The indications for laparoscopic pelvic lymph node dissection are still under discussion but, for cancer of the prostate, this procedure is certainly indicated before percutaneous high voltage therapy and before radical perineal prostatectomy. The siting of the ports, patient preparation and preoperative care have been described in detail by Schüssler et al.[31]

Major complications

Major complications during and after laparoscopic pelvic lymph node dissection requiring open surgical intervention can be expected in about 3–4% of cases.[32] The major complication rate could be even higher initially, depending on the learning curve of those urologists and urological institutions starting to undertake laparoscopic pelvic lymph node dissection.

Vascular injuries

The most commonly identified major complications of laparoscopic lymph node dissection are vascular injuries, with a frequency of about 1–1.5%. These may involve the epigastric artery owing to trocar placement, or the obturator veins, external and internal iliac arteries and external and internal iliac veins owing to careless lymph node dissection. Only about one-third of these vascular injuries require open surgical intervention; the other two-thirds can be handled by laparoscopic-guided fulguration, haemoclips and suture ligation. With increasing experience, the incidence of vascular injuries during pelvic lymphadenectomy is decreasing.

Ureteral injuries

Ureteral injuries, ranging from a small partial tear to complete ureteral transection, occur in particular after previous pelvic irradiation or after previous extensive surgery in this region. When ureteral injury is recognized during laparoscopic surgery an attempt can be made to insert a double-J stent transvesically and to adapt the ureteral tear by lap-aroscopic-guided sutures. A drainage tube should be placed in such cases for 3–4 days to prevent the development of urinomas. The authors successfully managed one ureteral tear, caused by lymph node dissection, by this means. However, where there is complete transection of the ureter or when a double-J stent is not available, an open repair should be performed immediately.

Bladder injuries

Bladder injuries due to trocar placement are noted mostly during laparoscopy and can be treated laparoscopically or by open repair. When the bladder injury is only small, a trial of catheter drainage alone is possible and should be followed by a cystogram after 9–10 days. Haematuria during or immediately after laparoscopic surgery, or signs of peritoneal irritation lasting more than 12 h after completion of lymph node dissection, should give rise to suspicion of an overlooked bladder injury.

Bowel injuries

Bowel injuries include perforation where the umbilical trocar passes through a bowel loop, and small bowel obstruction developing postoperatively due to herniation of the small intestine through a trocar site. The incidence of large bowel injuries is rare and is reported as 1–2.5 per thousand. When small bowel perforations are identified, laparoscopic repair can be considered; the safest approach, however, is always the open repair.

One of the most serious complications of laparoscopic surgery is the thermal bowel injury, when fulguration damages the bowel wall. Minor burns occurring as a result of adhesions in the small bony pelvis after previous irradiation or pelvic surgery may be followed by careful observation alone. Larger intestinal burn injuries must be explored immediately and bowel resection is commonly necessary. Unfortunately, bowel burn injuries are often not recognized until several days postoperatively with the symptoms of ileus or peritonitis. Abdominal pain and nausea in the first postoperative days always make an overlooked bowel injury suspect.

Minor complications

The incidence of post-laparoscopic lymphocoele is estimated at about 2% and compares favourably with open lymphadenectomy. Symptomatic or infected lymphocoeles after node dissection can be managed conservatively by percutaneous drainage with a Cystofix catheter until lymph production ceases after several days.

Fulguration of the obturator nerve can lead to transient or—after transection—to permanent weakness of the ipsilateral obturator muscle of the thigh.

Several other fairly minor complications, such as wound infections, prolonged scrotal swelling and urinary retention, developing after laparoscopic pelvic lymph node dissection, can be managed by observation alone in most cases and are not a problem in this procedure.

Conclusions

In connection with the discussion of complications during and after laparoscopic pelvic lymph node dissection, it must be asked whether the ability to detect positive nodes by laparoscopy is comparable to that with open dissection. To the author's knowledge, very few reports can answer this question. Winfield et al.[35] have reported their experience in a group of patients with laparoscopic lymph node dissection followed by open retropubic prostatectomy. There was one false negative in the laparoscopic group. Chodak et al.[36] attempted laparoscopic pelvic lymph node dissection in 18 cases followed by an open lymphadenectomy: 85% of lymph node metastases were detected by laparoscopy alone, whereas in two patients false-negative results occurred. These metastases were detected at the most proximal nodes of the internal iliac group, which might be difficult to reach laparoscopically.

At the time of writing—about 4 years after the introduction of laparoscopic lymph node dissection—an overall assessment of the relative merits of laparoscopic and open lymphadenectomy for the staging of prostate cancer seems appropriate.[37] Laparoscopic lymph node dissection is more time consuming than the surgical procedure; it is also more expensive and complications occur more frequently, whereas the hospital stay is shorter and the morbidity is lower. The ability to detect positive iliac and obturator lymph nodes by laparoscopy seems to be somewhat less than with open surgical lymphadenectomy, but will become equal with the increasing experience of the urologist. The well-known learning curve will reduce complications and will strengthen the place of laparoscopic pelvic lymph node dissection as an important and safe addition to the urological armamentarium for staging prostatic cancer in a specific group of patients. In the author's opinion, the indications for this procedure should be limited to patients below the age of 60 years, with extremely high risk factors for radical retropubic prostatectomy, to patients undergoing radiation therapy and to patients assigned for perineal prostatectomy. There is no place for performing laparoscopic lymph node dissection when a patient fulfils the criteria for a radical prostatectomy and the retropubic way is chosen. With these indications, laparoscopic pelvic lymph node dissection has an important place in the pretherapeutic staging of prostatic carcinomas and therefore also in the planning of curative therapeutic measures.

References

1. Sulmoni M, Jenny E, Müller J, Bandhauer K. Ureteroscopia per calcolosi ureterale: Indicazioni, agevolazioni tecniche, complicanze e risultati. Trib Med Ticinese 1994; 59: 276–278
2. Watson G. Mechanical and laser stone fragmentation in the ureter. Curr Opin Urol 1993; 3: 209–213
3. Anderson K R, Keetch D W, Albala D M et al. Optimal therapy for the distal ureter stone: extracorporeal shock wave lithotripsy versus ureteroscopy. J Urol 1994; 152: 62–65
4. Marberger M. Transurethral and transureteral stone manipulation. In: Marberger M,

Fitzpatrick J M, Jenkins A D, Pak C Y (eds) Stone surgery. Edinburgh: Churchill Livingstone, 1991; 115–166

5. Weinberg J J, Ansong K, Smith A D. Complications of ureteroscopy in relation to experience. J Urol 1987; 137: 384–387

6. Vicente J, Salvador J, Caparros J et al. Complicaciones de la ureteroscopia rigida. Actas Urol Esp 1991; 15: 55–58

7. Lyon E S, Huffman J L, Bagley D H. Ureteroscopic removal of upper tract calculi. In: Smith A D, Castaneda-Zuniga U R, Bronson J G (eds) Endourology principles and practice. Stuttgart: Thieme, 1986; 311–319

8. Daniels G F, Garnett J E Jr, Carter M F. Ureteroscopic results and complications: experience with 130 cases. J Urol 1988; 139: 710–713

9. Stackl W, Marberger M. Late sequelae of the management of ureteral calculi with the ureterorenoscope. J Urol 1986; 136: 386–389

10. Marberger M. Die Endoskopische Behandlung des Uretersteins. Urologe A 1984; 23: 308–316

11. Kramolowsky E V. Ureteral perforation during ureterorenoscopy: treatment and management. J Urol 1987; 138: 36–38

12. Rodrigues Netto N Jr, Caserta Lemos G, Levi D'Ancona C A et al. Is routine dilatation of the ureter necessary for ureteroscopy? Eur Urol 1990; 17: 269–272

13. Schwalb D M, Eshghi M, Davidian M, Franco I. Morphological and physiological changes in the urinary tract associated with ureteral dilation and ureteropyeloscopy: an experimental study. J Urol 1993; 149: 1576–1585

14. Camilleri J C, Schwalb D M, Eshghi M. Bilateral same session ureteroscopy. J Urol 1994; 152: 49–52

15. Wills T E, Burns J R. Ureteroscopy: an outpatient procedure. J Urol 1994; 151: 1185–1187

16. Motola J A, Badlani G H, Smith A D. Results of 212 consecutive endopyelotomies: an 8 year follow-up. J Urol 1993; 149: 453–456

17. Weiss J N, Badlani G H, Smith A D. Complications of endopyelotomy. Urol Clin North Am 1988; 15: 449–451

18. Korth K. Grenzen der perkutanen Steinchirurgie. Ergebnisse und neue Möglichkeiten des perkutanen Zuganges zur Niere. Urologe A 1984; 23: 302–307

19. Korth K, Künkel M, Ersching M. Perkutane Pyeloplastik. Urologe A 1987; 26: 173–180

20. Badlani G H, Karlin K S, Smith A D. Complications of endopyelotomy: analysis in series of 64 patients. J Urol 1988; 140: 473–475

21. Badlani G H, Eshghi M, Smith A D. Percutaneous surgery for ureteropelvic junction obstruction (endopyelotomy): technique and early results. J Urol 1986; 135: 26–28

22. Künkel M, Korth K. Langzeitergebnisse nach perkutaner Pyeloplastik. Urologe A 1990; 29: 325–329

23. Gerber G S, Lyon E S. Endourological management of upper tract urothelial tumors. J Urol 1993; 150: 2–7

24. Lim D J, Shattuck M C, Cook W A. Pyelovenous lymphatic migration of transitional cell carcinoma following flexible ureterorenoscopy. J Urol 1993; 149: 109–111

25. Kim J C, Banner M P, Ramchandani P et al. Balloon dilatation of ureteral strictures after renal transplantation. Radiology 1993; 186: 717–722

26. Flückiger F, Lammer J, Klein C E et al. Malignant ureteral obstruction—preliminary results of treatment with metallic self-expandable stents. Radiology 1993; 186: 169–173

27. Harding J R. Percutaneous antegrade ureteric stent insertion in malignant disease. J R Soc Med 1993; 86: 511–513

28. Coptcoat M J, Wickham J E. Laparoscopy in urology: current status. Eur Urol Update Ser 1992; 1: 58–63

29. Shichman S E J, Sosa E R. Frontiers in urology: laparoscopy. Curr Opin Urol 1993; 3: 214–219

30. Capelouto C C, Kavoussi L R. Complications of laparoscopic surgery. Urology 1993; 42: 2–12

31. Schüssler W W, Vancaillie T H G, Reich H, Griffith D P. Transperitoneal endosurgical lymphadenectomy in patients with localized prostate cancer. J Urol 1991; 145: 988–991

32. Kavoussi L R, Sosa E, Chandhoke P et al. Complications of laparoscopic pelvic lymph node dissection. J Urol 1993; 149: 322–325

33. Parra R O, Andrus C H, Boullier J A. Staging laparoscopic pelvic lymphnode dissection: experience and indications. Arch Surg 1992; 127: 1294–1297
34. Winfield H N, Schüssler W W. Pelvic lymphadenectomy: limited and extended. In: Clayman R V, McDougall E M (eds) Laparoscopic urology. St Louis: Quality Medical Publishing, 1993: 225–259.
35. Winfield H N, See W A, Donovan J F et al. Comparative effectiveness and safety of laparoscopic vs open pelvic lymph node dissection for cancer of the prostate. J Urol 1992; 147: 244A
36. Chodak G W, Levine L A, Gerber G S, Rukstalis D B. Safety and efficacy of laparoscopic lymphadenectomy. J Urol 1992; 147: 245A
37. Kerbl K, Clayman R, Petros J A et al. Staging pelvic lymphadenectomy for prostate cancer: a comparison of laparoscopic and open techniques. J Urol 1993; 150: 396–399

Urological complications of pelvic radiotherapy

4

E. Solsona   I. Iborra-Juan
J. V. Ricós-Torrent   J. L. Monrós-Lliso
R. Dumont-Martinez   J. L. Casanova-Ramon
J. López-Torrecilla

Radiobiological concepts

The efficacy of radiotherapy is well known in the treatment of malignant pelvic diseases, either as a single treatment or associated with chemotherapy or surgery. Its mechanism of action is not entirely clear, but it is known that DNA is the critical target of radiation, directly or indirectly through its interaction with the aqueous medium producing intermediary molecules that emit free radicals, The final effect is a molecular alteration in the DNA of the cell which, after one or more mitoses, loses its reproductive integrity, leading to its biological death.

If the irradiation dose is plotted against the probability of cure, a sigmoid curve is generated. The shape and slope of the curve depend on the following:

1. The intrinsic cellular radiosensitivity, which differs for each cellular species;
2. The dividing capacity of the cells, as it has been proved that the most sensitive cellular phases are the mitotic and G2 phases and the most resistant phases are G1 and, particularly, the S phase;
3. The cellular repair capacity, related to the non-lethal radiation cell damage according to the random effect of the ionizing radiation;
4. The environment of the cell, the most important factor being oxygen, in that oxygenated cells will be radiosensitive whereas hypoxic areas will be radioresistant.

These mechanisms are similar in both tumoral and normal tissues; thus the sigmoid curves for the tumour and for the normal tissues from which it is derived have the same characteristics, one corresponding to the tumour—the dose–response curve—and the other corresponding to the normal tissues—the dose-limiting curve. Therefore, the ideal dose (moderate probability of cure, low incidence of complications; Fig. 4.1, line a) is not the same as the optimal dose (high probability of cure, but increased incidence of complications; Fig. 4.1, line b) if the complication rate is taken into account. Much of the clinical investigation and research into the treatment of cancer is concerned with increasing the distance

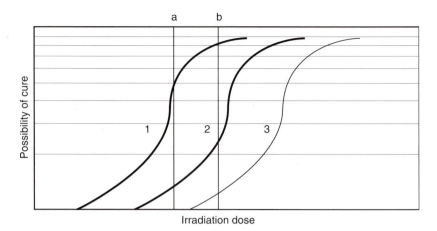

Figure 4.1. Irradiation dose versus probability of cure of malignant disease of the pelvis: curve 1, tumour dose–response curve; curve 2, incidence of major complications; curve 3, separated curve, i.e. altered incidence of complications, replacing curve 2; line a, 'ideal' dose; line b, 'optimal dose' (see text).

between these curves to reduce the complication rate for a given cure rate (curve 3; Fig. 4.1). With this aim, since the beginning of the 20th century the radiotherapy has been delivered in fractions.

Despite such fractionation, side effects are observed and they depend on the reproductive requirement of the cells to carry out their function. The acute effects are seen in frequently renewed tissues (high cell proliferation rate) such as the skin, mucosae and bone marrow; the late effects are observed in tissues with a low cell proliferation rate, such as the lung, nerves and muscle, these effects being, in fact, the dose-limiting factor. Two hypotheses to explain these delayed effects have been put forward: one attributes them to damage to the vasculoconnective stroma, whereas the other attributes them to damage to the endothelial cells, which are ubiquitous throughout the body.

All these effects result in the pathological processes of mucosal atrophy, the appearance of atypical fibroblasts in the submucosa and vascular changes such as vessel wall inelasticity, telangiectasia, and endothelial and myointimal proliferation, which lead to greater or lesser degrees of fibrosis and atypical neovascularization. These changes in the original irradiated tissues slowly and progressively develop into deeper lesions such as necrosis, fibrosis, fistulae and indolent ulcers.

Measures to prevent complications

Bearing in mind these radiobiological concepts, various technological measures have been taken in order to decrease the rate of complications after irradiation:

1. The acquisition of high-energy equipment (photons, electrons) has permitted more precise targeting of the radiation dose, with improved depth and avoidance of scatter, thus reducing the absorption by normal tissues;
2. New methods of interstitial radiotherapy, particularly in prostate cancer, with percutaneous perineal implantation under ultrasonographic control, has improved the geographical distribution of the implants;[1]
3. Three-dimensional planning and conformal radiotherapy, allowing a better definition of the area to be irradiated, has avoided unnecessary dosage of normal tissues, with promising preliminary results.[2,3]

Other measures, such as radioprotectors, heavy particles (heavy ions, protons, pi-mesons, neutrons), hyperbaric oxygen, hypoxic sensitizers (nitromidazole), DNA sensitizers with cytotoxic drugs (actinomycin D, doxorubicin, cisplatin), hyperthermia, hyperfractionation and the shrinking field and boost techniques, have not (yet) fulfilled their promise.

Another way of preventing complications may be to be aware of their predictive factors.[4-13] Despite controversy regarding the various predictive factors analysed in extended series of the Radiotherapy Oncology Group (RTOG) and the European Organization for the Research and Treatment of Cancer (EORTC), some have been considered to be predisposing factors. These include (a) the total dose: the risk is increased with doses higher than 55–60 Gy in bladder cancer, more than 70 Gy in prostate cancer and more than 85–90 Gy in gynecological cancer; (b) the target volume irradiated, and (c) previous surgery on the organs involved. Others seem to be more controversial: these include the duration of radiotherapy, previous acute complications, technical aspects (lateral, perineal boost), fractions higher than 2 Gy, pelvic geometry, diabetes, hypertension and age.

Literature review

In reviewing the literature for reported complications a series of problems has been found that impede analysis. These include the following:

1. The presence of different classifications [EORTC/RTOG, Chassagne glossary, ADDK (Århus, Denmark) system, personal classifications];
2. The absence of certain complications (incontinence, impotence) from some classifications;
3. Variation in the time at which complications are evaluated. Because of the evolutional character of the complication, a complication assessed as G2 could be G3 or G4 at a later evaluation;
4. Inclusion of complications requiring different medical or surgical treatment in the same group;
5. Failure to assess the morbidity resulting from the therapy required by such complications;

6. Difficulty in differentiating the aetiology of complications with regard to the culability of radiotherapy;
7. Differences in viewpoint of the various observers.

Despite these problems, radiotherapy, in general, showed a high rate of moderate complications (17.0–30.6%) but a fairly low rate of severe complications (6.1–8.3%), of major surgery required (1.1–7.6%) and of mortality due to complications (0.3–4.8%) (Table 4.1). The highest of these rates were in bladder cancer.[14–23] In prostate cancer, interstitial radiotherapy[1,24–30] involved a higher rate of severe complications, requirement for major surgery and mortality attributable to complications than external beam radiotherapy.[5,8,27,31–45] In gynaecological[6,7,46–58] and bowel cancer,[46,59–64] the complication rates were higher than in prostate cancer but the severe complications were mainly related to intestinal rather than to urological complications.

In this chapter, late and severe urological complications (G3, G4 and G5 of the RTOG/EORTC classification) are analysed, as these are the complications most often seen by urologists; however, other complications of particular interest are also discussed.

The severe urological complications associated with different malignant pelvic diseases treated with radiotherapy are summarized in Table 4.2.

Complications	Bladder cancer ($n = 2632$)	Prostate cancer†		Gynaecolog- ical cancer ($n = 9299$)	Bowel cancer ($n = 996$)
		External ($n = 6405$)	Interstitial ($n = 1791$)		
Moderate	20.7	19.3	30.6	17.0	18.1
	(4–32.1)	(4–74)	(14–50)	(10–27.4)	(16.2–22)
Severe	8.3	6.9	8.6	6.7	6.1
	(4–13.1)	(3–19)	(3–13.2)	(2–13)	(5.2–6.7)
Severe urological	5.1	4.7	20.3‡	4.6	1.1
	(3.8–8.2)	(1–9.4)	(9–32.2)	(1.5–11)	(0.5–1.8)
Severe intestinal	2.7	2.4	12.9‡	9.2	6.8
	(1.5–4.9)	(1–3.7)	(4.5–28.8)	(3.2–18.5)	(5–8.6)
Major surgery required	4.1	1.1	2.8	1.7	7.6§
	(1.2–7.3)	(0.2–2.1)	(2.2–3.2)	(1.4–3.1)	(4.9–13)
Complications mortality	4.8	0.3	1.2	2.9	1.2
	(1.2–7.3)	(0-0.7)	(0.5–6.3)	(0.5–5.0)	(0.6–2)

*Table 4.1. Complications of radiotherapy**

*Values are mean percentages, with ranges in parentheses.
†External, external beam radiotherapy; Interstitial, interstitial radiotherapy.
‡Moderate and severe complications.
§Bowel surgery.

Complications	Bladder cancer†		Prostate cancer†		Gynaecological cancer	Bowel cancer
	External	Interstitial	External	Interstitial		
Cystitis/ulcer	8.0	3.6	3.3	7.1	1.7	2.2
Bladder contracture	6.8	1.8	1.0	‡	‡	0.6
Haematuria	4.6	3.6	2.3	2.7	1.0	‡
Urethral stricture	‡	‡	4.7	7.3	—	—
Genital lymphoedema	‡		2.0	0.8	—	—
Incontinence	‡	5.2	4.0	2.7	0.3	1.2
Impotence	—	—	32.0	9.7	—	—
Bladder neck contracture	—	—	1.8	3.3	—	—
Prostate stricture	—	—	‡	2.2	—	—
Fistulae	‡	8.2	0.4	2.2	1.7	—
Ureteral stricture	‡	0.6	1.3	‡	1.3	0.5

Table 4.2. *Severe urological complications associated with malignant pelvic diseases treated with radiotherapy**

*Values are percentages.
†External, external beam radiotherapy; Interstitial, interstitial radiotherapy.
‡Uncommon.

In bladder cancer, complications are commonly located in the bladder. It is pointed out that an unincreased rate of bladder contracture (3.6%) but a slightly higher rate of cystectomies required (2.1%) were noted in 280 patients with a new therapy schedule associating transurethral resection (TUR), radiotherapy and systemic chemotherapy,[65–69] compared with radiotherapy alone (6.8 and 1.3%, respectively) (Table 4.3).

As Schellhammer and El-Mahdi[70] reported in a comparative non-randomized study, interstitial radiotherapy for prostate cancer has a greater urological complication rate than external beam radiotherapy; this was also confirmed, in general, in the present authors' review. With external beam radiotherapy, new perspectives have been opened, with the use of pre-liminary hormonal cytoreduction in an attempt to reduce the irradiated volume and thus increase the control of local disease and reduce the complication rate.[71,72]

Radiotherapy in gynaecological and rectosigmoid cancer has a low rate of severe urological complications; sometimes these are related to associated surgery.

Urological complications

Severe cystitis, bladder contracture and haematuria (Table 4.4)

These are the most frequent complications, being detected in all pelvic malignant pathologies irradiated, but the rate in bladder cancer is the highest. These complications appear to be related to total dose administered, to target volume and to previous bladder surgery.

In severe cystitis and bladder contracture to a capacity of more than 100–150 ml, the initial treatment should be conservative with anti-inflammatory and anti-spasmodic medication; if no remission occurs, orgotein, corticosteroids and (mainly) anticholinergic drugs may be given by systemic or endovesical administration, or both.[73,74] In the authors' experience, endovesical administration of hydrocortisone and oxybutin chloride has sometimes produced successful results. In extreme cases of cystitis or bladder contracture to a capacity of less than 100–150 ml, or when there is associated obstructive uropathy, radical cystectomy is the treatment of choice. This is the situation in 1.3–1.6% of cases; however, if there is no history of bladder cancer, a bladder reconstruction could be attempted.

Treatment of haematuria should take place in stages. Initial conservative treatment with systemic haemostatic agents, hyperbaric oxygen[75] and sodium pentosan polysulphate[76] has recently given encouraging results. Second, endovesical administration of aluminium salts[77,78] or glutaraldehyde[79] could be the first choice; if these fail, endovesical electrocoagulation of haemorrhagic sites or endovesical formalin could be the next option, but this last is not devoid of complications (renal insufficiency,

Treatment	No. of patients	Bladder contracture (%)	Cystectomy (%)
Rt* + chemotherapy	280	3.6	2.1
Rt alone	2643	6.8	1.3

Table 4.3. Rates of bladder contracture and cystectomy in patients undergoing transurethral resection of the prostate, given subsequent radiotherapy (Rt) plus chemotherapy, or chemotherapy alone
*Rt, radiotherapy.

peritonitis).[80,81] The Helmstein hydrostatic pressure technique[82] and selective embolization of anterior hypogastric branches[83] could be another choice. In the last stage, cystectomy is required in 0.2–1.2% of cases. Sometimes, cystectomy is not possible and a urinary diversion associated with hypogastric artery ligation may be performed, with controversial results,[81,84] or a high dose of endovesical formalin could be administered. In the authors' experience of 17 patients with severe haematuria after radiotherapy, endovesical aluminium salts followed by 4% formalin achieved a complete response with a haematuria-free interval of 108 days in 15 patients (88%); however, in 10 of these cases (67%) the haematuria recurred and nine patients (60%) required a more aggressive approach (Table 4.5).

Urethral stricture, bladder neck contracture, prostate stone, prostate stricture, impotence and incontinence (Table 4.6)

These complications occur almost exclusively in patients receiving radiotherapy for prostate cancer. They seem to be related to total radiation dose, irradiation portals, previous TUR and irradiation technique, being more frequent with interstitial radiotherapy (urethral, bladder neck and prostate strictures). Nevertheless, with external beam radiotherapy, impotence and incontinence are more frequent and may be related to vascular damage by irradiation, as reported by Goldstein and colleagues[85] and demonstrated by Doppler studies.

Urethral stricture usually responds well to dilatation or endoscopic urethrotomy, but in 0.2% of cases urethroplasty should be performed. Bladder neck contracture and prostate stricture can be alleviated with TUR or with bladder neck and prostate incision.

Ureteral obstruction and fistulae (Table 4.7)

Ureteral ostruction has a low prevalence (1.3%) when it is exclusively due to radiotherapy; however, more often it is associated with surgery or previous tumoral obstruction or recurrence, in which case the prevalence is markedly increased.[86] There is often a low rate of prostatorectal fistulae in prostate cancer, the rate being higher in interstitial radiotherapy than in

Complication: treatment	Bladder cancer†		Prostate cancer†		Gynaecological cancer	Bowel cancer
	External	Interstitial	External	Interstitial		
Severe cystitis:	8.0 (4.0–13.1)	3.6	3.3 (0.2–9.0)	7.1 (6–12.4)	1.7 (1.0–2.2)	2.2 (1.6–2.8)
cystectomy	1.6		0.5			
Bladder contracture:	6.8 (1.0–14.1)	1.8	1.0 (0.7–1.3)	‡	‡	0.6 (0.4–0.9)
surgery	1.3					
Haematuria:	4.6 (2.0–7.2)	3.6	2.3 (1.0–3.1)	2.7	1.0 (0.4–2.0)	‡
cystectomy	1.2				0.2	

Table 4.4. *Rates* of severe cystitis, bladder contracture and haematuria after radiotherapy of malignant diseases of the pelvis*

*Values are mean percentages, with ranges in parentheses.
†External, external beam radiotherapy; Interstitial, interstitial radiotherapy.
‡Uncommon.

Treatment	No. of patients
Cystectomy	2
Diversion + formalin (10%)	2
Percutaneous nephrostomy + formalin (10%)	3
None	1
Died of acute anaemia	1

Table 4.5. Final treatment of nine of 17 patients (53%) with severe haematuria after radiotherapy

external beam radiotherapy. In gynaecological cancer, fistulae are essentially vesicovaginal and, to a lesser extent, ureterovaginal or even more complex. The prevalence of these fistulae is markedly increased when the surgery is associated with radiotherapy.[87] Both complications are discussed in chapters 1 and 2.

Penoscrotal oedema

Penoscrotal oedema (Table 4.8) is preferentially related to prostatic irradiation, increasing in prevalence up to 20% when associated with pelvic lymphadenectomy;[28,29,43,88] however, only 0.3% of patients thus affected required surgical correction. In the authors' experience, removal of sclerolymphatic tissues and reconstruction with a free-skin graft results in a good aesthetic and functional solution.

Infertility

Infertility is another complication that involves all patients receiving pelvic irradiation, but it has special relevance to young patients, particularly to those with Hodgkin's disease and testicular seminoma who have received radiotherapy for the presence of pelvic lymph nodes or for prophylaxis. Despite protection of the testes with lead shields, the seminal cell line is involved: severe oligospermia was observed in most of the authors' patients but in 83% the sperm count was normal within an average of 26 months.

Second primary tumour

Patients with malignancy cured by radiotherapy have a higher risk of second primary tumour than the normal population. In patients with squamous cell carcinoma of the head and neck treated with radiotherapy the rate of second primary tumour was 15% at 5 years and 23% at 8 years; a similar trend has been observed in the upper respiratory and digestive tracts.[89] The appearance of secondary malignancies is directly related to the therapy modalities, the rate being higher when chemotherapy is associated.

In pelvic irradiation the risk is more debatable; sometimes the risk is greater in patients with benign pathologies than in those with irradiated neoplasia.

Complication: treatment	Bladder cancer†		Prostate cancer†		Gynaecological cancer	Bowel cancer
	External	Interstitial	External	Interstitial		
Urethral stricture: surgery	‡	‡	4.7 (1.0–9.1) 0.2	7.3 (1.1–9.4)	—	—
Bladder neck contracture	‡	—	1.8 (1.4–1.9)	3.3 (2.8–3.9)	—	—
Prostate stricture	—	—		2.2 (1.6–2.7)		
Incontinence	‡	5.2	4.0 (1.1–8.0)	2.7 (2.2–3.3)	0.3 (0.2–0.4)	1.2 (1.0–1.9)
Impotence	—	—	32.0 (10.0–41.0)	9.7 (7.2–25)	—	—

Table 4.6. Rates* of urethral stricture, bladder neck contracture, prostate stricture, incontinence and impotence after radiotherapy of malignant diseases of the pelvis

*Values are mean percentages, with ranges in parentheses.
†External, external beam radiotherapy; Interstitial, interstitial radiotherapy.
‡Uncommon.

Complication	Bladder cancer†		Prostate cancer†		Gynaecological cancer	Bowel cancer
	External	Interstitial	External	Interstitial		
Ureteral obstruction	‡	0.6	1.3 (0.4–2.7)	‡	1.3 (0.2–2.2)	0.5 (0.3–0.8)
Fistulae	‡	8.2	0.4 (0.0–2.2)	0.77 (2.7–4.4)	1.7 (0.1–5.0)	0.5 (0.3–0.8)

Table 4.7. Rates* of ureteral obstruction and fistulae

*Values are mean percentages, with ranges in parentheses.
†External, external beam radiotherapy; Interstitial, interstitial radiotherapy.
‡Uncommon.

Complication: treatment	Bladder cancer†		Prostate cancer†		Gynaecological cancer	Bowel cancer
	External	Interstitial	External	Interstitial		
Genital lymphoedema:	‡	—	2.0 (1.0–2.9)	0.8 (0.5–1)	—	—
surgery			0.3			

Table 4.8. Rates* of genital lymphoedema

*Values are mean percentages, with ranges in parentheses.
†External, external beam radiotherapy; Interstitial, interstitial radiotherapy.
‡Uncommon.

Surgical treatment of the complications

From 1.1 to 7.6% of patients receiving radiotherapy to the pelvis require major surgery because of the complications. Taking into account the radio-biological concepts mentioned above, some factors must be considered.

Salvage cystectomy is the most common surgical procedure, representing 16% of all irradiated patients with bladder cancer;[14,15,90–92] however, only 4.1% of such cases relate to complications of radiotherapy (Table 4.1). The morbidity and mortality rates for this procedure are higher than those for conventional cystectomy (Table 4.9). Urinary diversion is the main source of complications; for this reason, when surgery is recommended because of radiotherapy complications, ureteral section must be performed above the irradiation portal and, with regard to the bowel segment chosen, the trans-verse colon is to be preferred, as it is further from the field of irradiation. When salvage cystectomy is required because of recurrence of tumour, the factors predisposing to complications and the intestinal macroscopic aspect should be taken into account when selecting the bowel segment.

Other frequent surgical procedures on irradiated tissues relate to correction of fistulae. The interposition of revascularized tissues (omentum,[93] gracilis muscle[70,94] or seromuscular intestinal graft[95]) between the structures involved give a better chance of healing of the fistula. In the authors' experience of 12 cases of vesicovaginal fistula, one with ureterovesico vaginal fistula, attributable to interstitial and external irradiation associated with surgery, the interposition of omentum between bladder and vagina achieves healing in 100% of fistulae, leading to a 91% complete continence rate of 91%, with one patient with stress incontinence only.

Conclusions

1. The rates of severe urological complications, requirements for major surgery and mortality due to the complications arising from pelvic radiotherapy are fairly high. Given the new technological developments, this prevalence may be reduced.

2. The highest complication rate occurs in patients with irradiated bladder cancer. No significant increase in prevalence has been observed when radiotherapy is associated with transurethral resection and chemotherapy, but a longer follow-up is needed.

Cystectomy	Mortality	Complications	Fistulae	Reintervention
12.6	11.5	29.0	8.2	20.2
(7.7–18.8)	(0–24.3)	(14.3–42.1)	(2.0–11.3)	(18–20.9)

Table 4.9. Rates* of salvage cystectomy, mortality and morbidity in 535 patients receiving radiotherapy for bladder cancer

*Values are mean percentages, with ranges in parentheses.

3. Severe bladder complications are the most common and are sometimes difficult to resolve, requiring major surgery.

4. There are a great many complications associated with radiotherapy of prostate cancer, but the rates of requirement of major surgery and mortality due to complications are low, being higher after interstitial than after external beam radiotherapy. However, incontinence and impotence are markedly prevalent after external beam radiotherapy.

5. Initially, conservative measures may succeed; if they do not, however, complex surgical procedures may be necessary.

6. Surgical procedures on irradiated tissues have a high complication rate; radiobiological aspects should therefore be taken into account to decrease this rate. Such aspects include (a) those factors predisposing to complications, (b) the time at which surgery was performed, bearing in mind the evolutional nature of such complications, (c) the degree of irradiation of the tissues in relation to the siting of the irradiation portals, and (d) the possible use of revascularizing tissues.

7. In gynaecological and bowel cancer treated with radiotherapy, the rate of urological complications is low, but the prevalence is increased when surgery is associated. Fistulae are the most important complications observed.

8. Other complications, such as impairment of fertility and the appearance of a second malignancy, although occurring infrequently, should be taken into account when deciding on a course of therapy.

References

1. Brindle J S, Benson R C, Martinez A et al. Acute toxicity and preliminary therapeutic results of pelvic lymphadenectomy combined with transperineal interstitial implantation of 192IR and external beam radiotherapy for locally advanced prostate cancer. Urology 1985; 25: 233–238

2. Holm H H, Joul N, Pedersen J F et al. Transperineal 125-iodine seed implantation in prostatic cancer guided by transrectal ultrasonography. J Urol 1988; 140: 758–760

3. Vijayakumar S, Awan A, Karrison T et al. Acute toxicity during external-beam radiotherapy for localized prostate cancer: comparison of different techniques. Int J Radiat Oncol Biol Phys 1993; 25: 359–371

4. Crook J M, Esche B A, Chaplain G et al. Dose–volume analysis and the prevention of radiation sequelae in cervical cancer. Radiother Oncol 1987; 8: 321–332

5. Forman J D, Zinreich E, Lee D-J et al. Improving the therapeutic ratio of external beam irradiation for carcinoma of the prostate. Int J Radiat Oncol Biol Phys 1985; 11: 2073–2080

6. Hamberger A D, Unal A, Gershenson D M, Fletcher G H. Analysis of the severe complications of irradiation of carcinoma of the cervix: whole pelvis irradiation and intracavitary radium. Int J Radiat Oncol Biol Phys 1983; 9: 367–371

7. Hanks G E, Herring D F, Kramer S. Patterns of care outcome studies. Cancer 1983; 51: 959–967

8. Mameghan H, Fisher R, Mameghan J et al. Bowel complications after radiotherapy for carcinoma of the prostate: the volume effect. Int J Radiat Oncol Biol Phys 1990; 18: 315–320

9. Nussbaum H, Kagan A R, Wollin M et al. Guidelines for radiation injury to bowel and bladder from external irradiation alone. Cancer Clin Trials 1981; 4: 295–299

10. Orton C G. Dose dependence of complication rates in cervix cancer radiotherapy. Int J Radiat Oncol Biol Phys 1986; 12: 37–44

11. Perez C A, Fox S, Lockett M A et al. Impact of dose in outcome of irradiation alone in carcinoma of the uterine cervix: analysis of two different methods. Int J Radiat Oncol Biol Phys 1991; 21: 885–898

12. Pilepich M V, Perez C A, Walx B J, Zivnuska F R. Complications of definitive radiotherapy for carcinoma of the prostate. Int J Radiat Oncol Biol Phys 1981; 7: 1341

13. Seymore C H, El-Mahdi A M, Schellhammer P F. The effect of prior transurethral resection of the prostate on post radiation urethral strictures and bladder neck contractures. Int J Radiat Oncol Biol Phys 1986; 12: 1597–1600

14. Blandy J P, England H R, Evans S J W et al. T3 bladder cancer—the case for salvage cystectomy. Br J Urol 1980; 52: 506–510

15. Corcoran M O, Thomas D M, Lim A et al. Invasive bladder cancer treated by radical external radiotherapy. Br J Urol 1985; 57: 40–42

16. Goodman G B, Hislop G, Elwood J M, Balfour J. Conservation of bladder function in patients with invasive bladder cancer treated by definitive irradiation and selective cystectomy. Int J Radiat Oncol Biol Phys 1981; 7: 569–573

17. Hewitt C B, Babiszewski J F, Antunez A R. Update on intracavitary radiation in the treatment of bladder tumors. J Urol 1981; 126: 323–325

18. Mameghan H, Fisher R. Invasive bladder cancer. Prognostic factors and results of radiotherapy with and without cystectomy. Br J Urol 1989; 63: 251–258

19. Quilty P M, Duncan W, Chisholm G D et al. Results of surgery following radical radiotherapy for invasive bladder cancer. Br J Urol 1986; 58: 396–405

20. Van Der Werf-Messing B, Hop W C J. Carcinoma of the urinary bladder (Category T1,Nx,M0) treated either by radium implant or by transurethral resection only. Int J Radiat Oncol Biol Phys 1981; 7: 299–303

21. Van Der Werf-Messing B H P. Cancer of the urinary bladder treated by interstitial radium implant. Int J Radiat Oncol Biol Phys 1978; 4: 373–378

22. Williams G B, Trott P A, Bloom H J G. Carcinoma of the bladder treated by interstitial irradiation. Br J Urol 1981; 53: 221–224

23. Yu W S, Sagerman R H, Chung C H et al. Experience with radical and preoperative radiotherapy in 421 patients. Cancer 1985; 56: 1293-1299

24. Carlton C E, Scardino P T. Combined interstitial and external irradiation for prostatic cancer. In: Murphy G, Khoury S, Chatelain C, Denis L (eds) Prostate cancer in questions. New York: Liss, 1992; 63–66

25. Fowler J E, Barzell W, Hilaris B S, Whitmore W F. Complications of 125-iodine implantation and pelvic lymphadenectomy in the treatment of prostatic cancer. J Urol 1979; 121: 447–451

26. Lannon S G, El-Araby A A, Joseph P K et al. Long-term results of combined interstitial gold seed implantation plus external beam irradiation in localised carcinoma of the prostate. Br J Urol 1993; 72: 782–791

27. Schellhammer P F, Whitmore R B, Kuban D A et al. Morbidity and mortality of local failure after definitive therapy for prostate cancer. J Urol 1989; 141: 567–571

28. Sommerkamp H. Pelvic lymphadenectomy and brachytherapy for prostatic cancer. Eur Urol 1986; 12: 265–269

29. Whitehead E D, Huh S H, Garcia R L et al. Interstitial irradiation of carcinoma of the prostate with 125-iodine and simultaneous extraperitoneal pelvic lymphadenectomy in 32 patients: trials, tribulations and possible triumphs. J Urol 1981; 126: 366–371

30. Whitmore W F, Hilaris B, Sogani P et al. Interstitial irradiation using I-125 seeds. In: Murphy G, Khoury S, Chatelain C, Denis L (eds) Prostate cancer in questions. New York: Liss, 1992; 59–62

31. Bagshaw M A, Ray G R, Cox R S. Radiation technique. In: Murphy G, Khoury S, Chatelain C, Denis L (eds) Prostate cancer in questions. New York: Liss, 1992; 54–55

32. Benk V A, Adams J A, Shipley W U et al. Late rectal bleeding and proton high dose irradiation for patients with stages T3–T4 prostate carcinoma. Int J Radiat Oncol Biol Phys 1993; 26: 551–557

33. Douchez J, Allain Y M, Cellier P et al. Cancer de la prostate: intolerance et morbidité de la radiothérapie externe. Bull Cancer (Paris) 1985; 72: 573–577

34. Gibbons R P, Tate Mason J, Correa R J et al. Carcinoma of the prostate: local control with external beam radiation therapy. J Urol 1979; 121: 310–312

35. Green N, Goldberg H, Goldman H et al. Severe rectal injury following radiation for prostatic cancer. J Urol 1984; 131: 701–704
36. Hafermann M D, Gibbons R P, Murphy G P. Quality control of radiation therapy in multi-institutional randomized clinical trial for localized prostate cancer. Urology 1988; 31: 119–124
37. Hanks G E, Krall J M, Martz K L et al. The outcome of treatment of 313 patients with T-1 (UICC) prostate cancer treated with external beam irradiation. Int J Radiat Oncol Biol Phys 1988; 14: 243–248
38. Kurup P, Kramer T S, Lee M S, Phillips R. External beam irradiation of prostatic cancer. Cancer 1984; 53: 37–43
39. Lai P P, Perez C A, Shapiro S J, Lockett M A. Carcinoma of the prostate state B and C: lack of influence of duration of radiotherapy on tumor control and treatment morbidity. Int J Radiat Oncol Biol Phys 1990; 19: 561–568
40. Lawton C A, Won M, Pilepich M V et al. Long-term treatment sequelae following external beam irradiation for adenocarcinoma of the prostate: analysis of RTOG Studies 7506 and 7706. Int J Radiat Oncol Biol Phys 1991; 21: 935–939
41. Lindholt J, Hansen P T. Prostatic carcinoma: complications of megavoltage radiation therapy. Br J Urol 1986; 58: 52–54
42. Read G, Pointon R C S. Retrospective study of radiotherapy in early carcinoma of the prostate. Br J Urol 1989; 63: 191–195
43. Schubert J, Kelly L U, Wehnert J, Moravek P. Radical pelvic surgery and radiation therapy in the management of localized carcinoma of the prostate. Eur Urol 1988; 14: 196–201
44. Smit W G J M, Helle P A, Van Putten W L J et al. Late radiation damage in prostate cancer patients treated by high dose external radiotherapy in relation to rectal dose. Int J Radiat Oncol Biol Phys 1990; 18: 23–29
45. Zagars G K, Von Eschenbach A C, Johnson D E, Oswald M J. Stage C adenocarcinoma of the prostate. Cancer 1987; 60: 1489–1499
46. Dean R J, Lytton B. Urologic complications of pelvic irradiation. J Urol 1978; 119: 64–67
47. Gerbaulet A L, Kunkler I H, Kerr G R et al. Combined radiotherapy and surgery: local control and complications in early carcinoma of the uterine cervix—the Villejuif experience, 1975–1984. Radiother Oncol 1992; 23: 66–73
48. Greven K M, Lanciano R M, Herbert S H, Hogan P E. Analysis of complications in patients with endometrial carcinoma receiving adjuvant irradiation. Int J Radiat Oncol Biol Phys 1991; 21: 919–923
49. Horiot J-C, Pigneux J, Pourquier H et al. Radiotherapy alone in carcinoma of the intact uterine cervix according to G. H. Fletcher guidelines:-a French cooperative study of 1383 cases. Int J Radiat Oncol Biol Phys 1988; 14: 605–611
50. Kjorstad K E, Martimbeau P W, Iversen T. Stage IB carcinoma of the cervix, the Norwegian radium hospital: results and complications. Gynaecol Oncol 1983; 15: 42–47
51. Montana G S, Fowler W C. Carcinoma of the cervix: analysis of bladder and rectal radiation dose and complications. Int J Radiat Oncol Biol Phys 1989; 16: 95–100
52. Okawa T, Kita M, Goto M, Tazaki E. Radiation therapy alone in the treatment of carcinoma of the uterine cervix: review of experience at Tokyo women's medical college (1969–1983). Int J Radiat Oncol Biol Phys 1987; 13: 1845–1849
53. Pedersen D, Bentzen S M, Overgaard J. Reporting radiotherapeutic complications in patients with uterine cervical cancer. The importance of latency and classification system. Radiother Oncol 1993; 28: 134–141
54. Perez C A, Breaux S, Bedwinek J M et al. Radiation therapy alone in the treatment of carcinoma of the uterine cervix. Cancer 1984; 54: 235–246
55. Sinistrero G, Sismondi P, Rumore A, Zola P. Analysis of complications of cervix carcinoma treated by radiotherapy using the Franco-Italian glossary. Radiother Oncol 1993; 26: 203–211
56. Strockbine M F, Hancock J E, Fletcher G H. Complications in 831 patients with squamous cell carcinoma of the intact uterine cervix treated with 3,000 rads or more whole pelvis irradiation. Am J Roentgenol 1970; 108: 293–304
57. Stryker J A, Bartholomew M, Velkley D E et al. Bladder and rectal complications following radiotherapy for cervix cancer. Gynecol Oncol 1988; 29: 1–11
58. Tak W K, Munzenrider J E, Mitchell G W. External irradiation and one radium application for carcinoma of the cervix. Int J Radiat Oncol Biol Phys 1979; 5: 29–36

59. Mak A C, Rich T A, Schulteiss T E et al. Late complications of postoperative radiation therapy for cancer of the rectum and rectosigmoid. Int J Radiat Oncol Biol Phys 1994; 28: 597–603

60. Krook J E, Moertel C G, Gunderson L L et al. Effective surgical adjuvant therapy for high-risk rectal carcinoma. N Engl J Med 1991; 324: 709–715

61. Sparso B H, Von Der Maase H, Kristensen D et al. Complications following postoperative combined radiation and chemotherapy in adenocarcinoma of the rectum and rectosigmoid. Cancer 1984; 54: 2363–2366

62. Tepper J E, Cohen A M, Wood W C et al. Postoperative radiation therapy of rectal cancer. Int J Radiat Oncol Biol Phys 1987; 13: 5–10

63. Thomas P R M, Lindblad A S, Stablein D M et al. Toxicity associated with adjuvant postoperative therapy for adenocarcinoma of the rectum. Cancer 1986; 57: 1130–1134

64. Vigliotti A, Rich T A, Romsdahl M M et al. Postoperative adjuvant radiotherapy for adenocarcinoma of the rectum and rectosigmoid. Int J Radiat Oncol Biol Phys 1987; 13: 999–1006

65. Cervek J, Cufer T, Krageli B et al. Sequential transurethral surgery, multiple drug chemotherapy and radiation therapy for invasive bladder carcinoma: initial report. Int J Radiat Oncol Biol Phys 1993; 25: 777–782

66. Jarse G, Frommhold H, Zur Nedden D. Combined radiation and chemotherapy for locally advanced transitional cell carcinoma of the urinary bladder. Cancer 1985; 55: 1659–1664

67. Kubota Y, Shuin T, Miura T et al. Treatment of bladder cancer with a combination of hyperthermia, radiation and bleomycin. Cancer 1984; 53: 199–202

68. Tester W, Porter A, Asbell S et al. Combined modality program with possible organ preservation for invasive bladder carcinoma: results of RTOG PROTOCOL 85–12. Int J Radiat Oncol Biol Phys 1993; 25: 783–790

69. Zietman A L, Shipley W U, Kaufman D S. The combination of cis-platin based chemotherapy and radiation in the treatment of muscle-invading transitional cell cancer of the bladder. Int J Radiat Oncol Biol Phys 1993; 27: 161–170

70. Schellhammer P F, El-Mahdi A M. Pelvic complications after definitive treatment of prostate cancer by interstitial or external beam radiation. Urology 1993; 21: 451–457

71. Pilepich M V, Krall J M, John M J et al. Hormonal cytoreduction in locally advanced carcinoma of the prostate treated with definitive radiotherapy: preliminary results of RTOG 83-07. Int J Radiat Oncol Biol Phys 1989; 16: 813–817

72. Shearer R J, Davies J H, Gelister J S K, Dearnaley D P. Hormonal cytoreduction and radiotherapy for carcinoma of the prostate. Br J Urol 1992; 69: 521–524

73. Kato K, Kondo A, Saito M et al. In vitro intravesical oxybutynin chloride in children with neurogenic bladder. J Urol 1991; 47: 36–38

74. Prasad K V R, Vaidyanathan S. Intravesical oxybutynin chloride and clean intermittent catheterisation in patients with neurogenic vesical dysfunction and decreased bladder capacity. Br J Urol 1993; 72: 719–722

75. Weiss J P, Mattel D M, Hanno P M. Hyperbaric oxygen treatment of radiation-induced hemorrhagic cystitis: ten years experience. J Urol 1994; 151: 378A (abstr 602)

76. Hampson S J, Woodhouse C R J. Sodium pentosan polysulphate in the management of hemorrhagic cystitis due to radiation damage. Experience with 14 patients. J Urol 1993; 149: 489A (abstr 1107)

77. Arrizabalaga M, Extramiana J, Parra J L et al. Treatment of massive haematuria with aluminous salts. Br J Urol 1987; 60: 223–226

78. Ostroff E B, Chenault O W. Alum irrigation for the control of massive bladder hemorrhage. J Urol 1982; 128: 929–930

79. Gastón de Iriarte E, Martínez-Piñeiro J A, De la Pena J et al. La hemorragia vesical incoercible. 'Gluteraldehización', nueva alternativa terapéutica? Actas Urol Esp 1981; 5: 353–358

80. Brown R B. A method of management of inoperable carcinoma of the bladder. Med J Aust 1969; 1: 23–26

81. McGuire E J, Weiss R M, Schiff M, Lytton B. Hemorrhagic radiation cystitis. Urology 1974; 3: 204–208

82. Helmstein K. Treatment of bladder carcinoma by a hydrostatic pressure technique. Br J Urol 1972; 44: 434

83. Appleton D S, Sibley G N A, Doyle P T. Internal iliac artery embolisation for the control of severe bladder and prostate haemorrhage. Br J Urol 1988; 61: 45–47

84. Le Guillou M, Merland J J, Lepage T et al. Controle des hématuries vésicales incoercibles par embolisation vésicale sélective: 7 observations de cystites radiques et de tumeurs récidivées. Nouv Presse Med 1975; 4: 1703–1707

85. Goldstein I, Feldman M, Deckers P J et al. Radiation-associated impotence: a clinical study of its mechanism. JAMA 1984; 251: 903

86. Bahrassa F, Ampil F. Posttreatment ureteral obstruction in invasive carcinoma of uterine cervix. Int J Radiat Oncol Biol Phys 1987; 13: 23–28

87. Weems D H, Mendenhall W M, Bova F J et al. Carcinoma of the intact uterine cervix, stage IB-IIIA-B > /=6 cm in diameter: irradiation alone vs preoperative irradiation and surgery. Int J Radiat Oncol Biol Phys 1985; 11: 1911–1914

88. Greskovich F J, Zagars G K, Sherman N E, Johnson D E. Complications following external beam radiation therapy for prostate cancer: an analysis of patients treated with and without staging pelvic lymphadenectomy. J Urol 1991; 146: 798–802

89. Cooper J S, Pajak T F, Rubin P et al. Second malignancies in patients who have head and neck cancers: incidence, effect on survival and implications based on the RTOG experience. Int J Radiat Oncol Biol Phys 1989; 17: 449–456

90. Abratt R P, Wilson J A, Pontin A R, Barnes R D. Salvage cystectomy after radical irradiation for bladder cancer—prognostic factors and complications. Br J Urol 1993; 72: 756–760

91. Johnson D E. Salvage cystectomy. Semin Urol 1983; 1: 53–59

92. Smith J A, Whitmore W F. Salvage cystectomy for bladder cancer after failure of definitive irradiation. J Urol 1981; 125: 643–645

93. Mraz J P, Sutory M. Alternative in surgical treatment of post-irradiation vesicovaginal and rectovaginal fistulas: seromuscular intestinal graft (patch). J Urol 1994; 151: 357–359

94. Menchaca A, Akhyat M, Gleicher N et al. The rectus abdominis muscle flap in a combined abdominovaginal repair of difficult vesicovaginal fistulae. A report of three cases. J Reprod Med 1990; 35: 565–568

95. Turner-Warwick R T, Wynne E J C, Handley-Ashken M. The use of the omental pedicle graft in the repair and reconstruction of the urinary tract. Br J Surg 1967; 54: 849–853

Management of radiation-induced vesicovaginal fistulae

5

N. K. Bissada

Introduction

In patients who have received preoperative radiation therapy and who develop vesicovaginal fistula after radical surgery, the fistula may be repaired in standard fashion provided that the tissues are well vascularized. Wisdom dictates the placement of intervening non-irradiated tissue between the bladder and vaginal closure.

When fistulization occurs as a result of radiation necrosis, local tissues are usually unsuitable for repair. They never close spontaneously. The surrounding tissues are fibrotic, inelastic, and with poor vascularity as a result of radiation-induced endarteritis obliterans. These are truly radiation-induced vesicovaginal fistulae, and are among the most difficult urological problems to manage.[1,2] Successful repair requires increasing vascularity at the fistula site by mobilizing vascular pedicles. Several vascular pedicles have been used for this purpose, including the gluteus maximus, adductor longus, gracilis, sartorius, rectus abdominis, pubococcygeus and bulbocavernosus muscles, labial fat pad, stomach and omentum.[2–10]

Before attempting repair, recurrent malignancy must be ruled out by biopsy. Generally, repair should be delayed long enough to allow demarcation and slough of necrotic tissue with stabilization of the fistula.

Most radiation-induced vesicovaginal fistulae that are suitable for primary repair and are not associated with ureteral or bowel involvement may be repaired vaginally. This has the advantage of obviating the need for bowel manipulation in a previously irradiated field if an abdominal approach is used. Currently, with a vaginal approach, the most frequently used tissues for interposition are the Martius flap and the gracilis muscle flap. If it is necessary to use an abdominal approach, the omentum[1,11] or a combination of gastric and omental segments based on the gastroepiploic vessels is most suitable for interposition.

Although colpocleisis has been advocated by some, in the author's opinion it is associated with a number of problems that discourage its use.[5,12]

Modified Martius flap techniques

The Martius flap technique involves mobilization of the bulbocavernosus muscle and labial fat pad.[1,13,14] This technique and several modifications of it have become the author's preferred techniques because of their simplicity and effectiveness. Because of the frequent presence of extensive scarring, a generous episiotomy at the 5 or 7 o'clock position may be required. This divides the pubococcygeus and transverse perineal muscles and a portion of the levator ani muscle. Once adequate exposure has been obtained, the fistula is excised and the bladder and vaginal walls are mobilized. The mobilization needs to be more generous than in non-irradiated fistulae in order to allow closure without tension. The bladder is closed with 3/0 polyglycolic acid sutures. Subsequently, the skin of the medial aspect of the labium major on the contralateral side to the episiotomy is incised vertically from the level of the mons pubis to the lower third of the labium. The skin edges are mobilized and retracted (Fig. 5.1a). The Martius flap consists of the bulbocavernosus muscle and its labial fat pad. This is exposed and dissected. The Martius flap is divided high at the level of the mons pubis to provide sufficient length to reach and cover the fistula without tension (Fig. 5.1b). A tunnel is then formed under the skin between the labium major and the fistula, through the lateral vaginal wall. The tunnel must be wide enough to prevent compression of the blood supply to the pedicle. The flap is passed through the tunnel and placed over the closed bladder defect. The Martius flap completely covers the bladder closure and is anchored in place with 3/0 polyglycolic acid sutures (Fig. 5.1c). The vaginal mucosa is then closed over the pedicle.

Often there is not enough vaginal mucosa to close the defect. The muscle will become completely epithelialized. The author's preference, however, is to cover the defect with a myocutaneous flap, as described and illustrated in Fig. 5.2a–c.

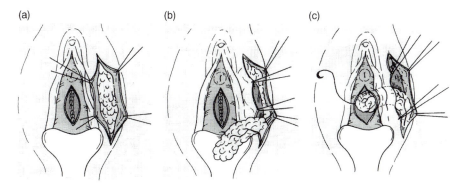

Figure 5.1. Martius flap technique. (a) Bladder closed. Bulbocavernosus muscle–labial fat pad exposed through a medial labial incision. (b) Martius flap raised. Pedicle based posteriorly. (c) The Martius flap is passed through a generous tunnel to the site of the fistula. The distal part of the Martius flap completely covers the fistula and is sutured to the underlying tissue. Vaginal wall is closed over the Martius flap without tension. If there is no adequate vaginal tissue to close over the defect without tension, the graft may be left uncovered and will become completely epithelialized. Preferably, the technique shown in Figs 2a–c may be used. (Reproduced from ref. 1 with permission.)

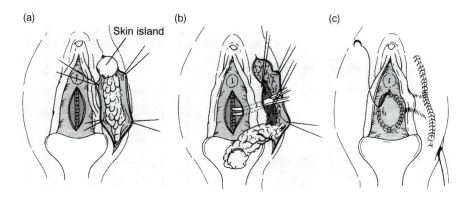

Figure 5.2. Myocutaneous graft technique. (a) When the surgeon anticipates that vaginal mucosa will be inadequate to close over the Martius flap, an island skin graft may be created together with the Martius fibrofatty–bulbocavernosus muscle flap (myocutaneous graft). The bladder has been closed. The Martius flap is exposed through a labial incision. The skin island is outlined over the distal part of the flap. (b) The skin island is separated from surrounding skin but is left attached to the mobilized Martius flap. It is anchored to the underlying fibrofatty tissue with fine absorbable sutures to prevent incidental shearing of the skin from underlying tissue. A tunnel is created between the labial incision and the site of the fistula. (c) The flap is passed through the tunnel. The island skin graft is sutured to the surrounding vaginal mucosa, completely covering the defect. The labial incision is closed after placing a Penrose drain. (Reproduced from ref. 1 with permission.)

The author has also used double island myocutaneous skin flaps, as described and illustrated in Fig. 5.3a,b.

If an episiotomy has been performed, it is then closed with absorbable sutures after placing a small Penrose drain. The labial incision is also closed

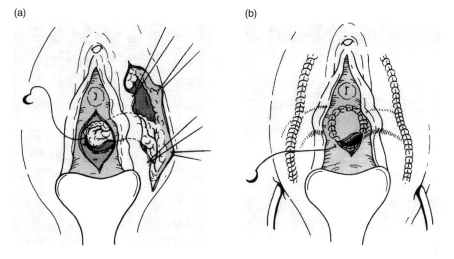

Figure 5.3. Double island flaps. (a) An island myocutaneous bulbocavernosus flap is created as in Fig. 5.2. It is rotated and the skin island is anastomosed to the bladder edges. (b) The skin island of the contralateral myocutaneous flap is sutured to the vaginal edges to cover the vaginal defect. (Reproduced from ref. 1 with permission.)

with absorbable sutures after placing a small Penrose drain. The drains are removed at 48 h postoperatively.

Gracilis muscle flap technique

Several authors have advocated the use of gracilis muscle brought from one or both sides for interposition between bladder and vaginal closures.[15–17] The technique is similar to that described above, except for the use of a gracilis pedicle instead of a Martius flap. For obtaining a gracilis pedicle an incision is made overlying the course of the gracilis muscle. The muscle flap is developed. The gracilis is divided at the medial femoral condyle and is dissected free in a cephalad direction. The blood supply is encountered about 8–10 cm from its origin and should not be disturbed. A tunnel is developed between the thigh and the fistula site. The distal end of the muscle flap is passed through the tunnel and anchored to the pubocervical fascia along the opposite margin of the defect with 3/0 polyglycolic acid sutures so that the muscle completely covers the bladder closure. Vaginal closure is performed as described above.

Use of combined gastric and omental segments

Through a midline transperitoneal approach the bladder is exposed and opened. The ureters are catheterized. The bladder incision is extended to the fistula. The fistula is widely excised, removing all apparent non-vascularized and necrotic or fibrotic tissue. If the vagina is markedly scarred, it may be impossible to close without tension; in this case the gap is closed by a vascularized omental segment and the bladder defect is closed with the gastric segment.[2] It is crucial to ensure adequate blood supply to the segments by routine testing of the patency of the left and right gastroepiploic vessels before selecting the side to be used as a pedicle for the gastric and omental segments.[18] The gastric segment is outlined on the anterior and posterior walls with the base at the greater curvature. The segment is separated from the stomach and the stomach continuity is re-established. The omental flap is also isolated. The gastroepiploic vessels are mobilized off the stomach to create an adequate pedicle (Fig. 5.4). The combined stomach and omentum segments are both based on the same pedicle and are brought down to the site of the fistula. The omental patch is used either to bridge the vaginal defect or as an interposition between the vaginal closure posteriorly and the gastrocystoplasty anteriorly. The gastric segment is sutured to the bladder, replacing the posterior bladder wall. The anterior bladder wall is approximated. The bladder is decompressed with a suprapubic tube as well as an indwelling urethral catheter for 3–4 weeks. Indwelling ureteric catheters are optional. Sexual intercourse is prohibited for 3 months.

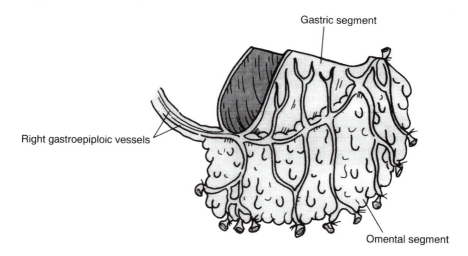

Figure 5.4. Combined gastric and omental segments based on the gastroepiploic vessels. The omental segment is used either to bridge the vaginal defect or as an interposition graft between the vaginal closure posteriorly and the bladder anteriorly. The gastric segment is sutured to the fresh edges of the bladder to replace the posterior bladder wall.

Results and conclusions

As stated earlier, patients who previously received radiation therapy and who develop vesicovaginal fistula can be anticipated to have excellent results with proper surgical techniques.[19,20] On the other hand, the cure of radiation-induced vesicovaginal fistula is not nearly as good.[1,3,21] In the author's experience with 28 such patients, only ten were suitable for primary repair. Successful closure was accomplished in nine of these ten patients (90%). Ten other patients were judged not suitable for primary repair and underwent supravesical diversion. The risk of using irradiated lower ureter and bowel must be considered in these patients. The author prefers a transverse colon conduit as the most suitable for conduit diversion. For continent urinary diversion, the Charleston pouch has been used initially in these patients.[22] However, currently the author recommends a non-radiated gastrocolic pouch when continent diversion is performed in patients with radiation-induced vesicovaginal fistulae.[23]

Some patients will be unsuitable for any surgical management. These must be managed with supportive non-operative palliative measures.

This experience indicates that patients with radiation-induced vesicovaginal fistulae represent a heterogeneous group, and that careful assessment, proper selection, timing and choice of appropriate surgical procedures are crucial. However, with adherence to these guidelines, most of them can be managed satisfactorily.

References

1. Bissada N K. Genitourinary fistulas. In: Rous S N (ed) Urology annual. Norwalk, Appleton and Lange, 1991; 5: 115–149
2. Bissada S A, Bissada N K. Repair of active radiation-induced vesicovaginal fistula using combined gastric and omental segments based on the gastroepiploic vessels. J Urol 1992; 147: 1368–1370
3. Boronow R C. Repair of the radiation-induced vaginal fistula utilizing the Martius technique. World J Surg 1986; 10: 237–248
4. McCall M L, Bolten K A. Martius' Gynecological operations. Boston: Little, Brown, 1956; 327
5. Boronow R C, Rutledge F. Vesicovaginal fistula, radiation and gynecologic cancer. Am J Obstet Gynecol 1971; 111: 85
6. Bastiaanse N A, Van B. Bastiaanse's method for surgical closure of very large irradiation fistula of the bladder and rectum. In: Youssef A F (ed) Gynecological urology. Springfield: Charles C. Thomas, 1960.
7. Graham J B. Vaginal fistulas following radiotherapy. Surg Gynecol Obstet 1965; 120: 1019
8. Byron R L, Ostergard D R. Sartorius muscle interposition for the radiation-induced vaginal fistula. Am J Obstet Gynecol 1969; 104: 104
9. Stirnemann H. Treatment of recurrent recto-vaginal fistula by interposition of a gluteus maximus muscle flap. Am J Proctol 1969; 20: 52
10. Buchsbaum H J, Schmidt J D, Platz C et al. Radiation cystitis, fistula and fibrosis. In: Buchsbaum H J, Schmidt J D (eds) Gynecologic and obstetric urology. Philadelphia: Saunders, 1978; 275–297
11. Kiricuta I, Goldstein A M B. The repair of extensive vesicovaginal fistulas with pedicled omentum: a review of 27 cases. J Urol 1972; 108: 724–727
12. Boronow R C. Urologic complications secondary to radiation alone or radiation and surgery. In: Delgado G, Smith J P (eds) Management of complications in gynecologic oncology. New York: Wiley, 1982: 163–197
13. Hoskins W J, Park R C, Long R et al. Repair of urinary tract fistulas with bulbocavernosus myocutaneous flaps. Obstet Gynecol 1984; 63: 588
14. Patil U, Waterhouse K, Laungani G. Management of 18 difficult vesicovaginal and urethrovaginal fistulas with modified Ingleman–Sunberg and Martius operations. J Urol 1980; 123: 653–656
15. Obrink A, Bunne G. Gracilis interposition in fistulas following radiotherapy for cervical cancer: a retrospective study. Urol Int 1978; 33: 370
16. Ryan J A Jr, Gibbons R P, Correa R J Jr. Urologic use of gracilis muscle flap for non-healing perineal wounds and fistulas. Urology 1985; 26: 456–459
17. Fleischman J, Picha G. Abdominal approach for gracilis muscle interposition and repair of recurrent vesicovaginal fistulas. J Urol 1988; 140: 552–554
18. Bissada S A, Bissada N K. Choice of gastroepiploic vessels for gastrocystoplasty. J Urol 1992; 148: 101
19. Bissada N K, McDonald D. Management of giant vesicovaginal and vesicourethrovaginal fistulas. J Urol 1983; 130: 1073–1075
20. Bissada N K, Morcos R R. Voiding patterns and urinary control after repair of giant vesicovaginal and vesicourethrovaginal fistulas and neourethral construction. Neurourol Urodynam 1986; 5: 321–323
21. Zimmern P E, Hadley H R, Staskin D R et al. Genitourinary fistulae: vaginal approach for repair of vesicovaginal fistulae. Urol Clin North Am 1985; 12: 361–367
22. Bissada N K. New continent urinary reservoir: Charleston pouch with minimally altered in-situ appendix. Urology 1993; 41: 524–526
23. Kaczmareck T, Bissada N K. New gastrocolic urinary reservoir with gastric tube outlet: experimental and clinical experience. J Urol 1995; 153: 242A

Severe urinary tract damage following radiotherapy for cervical carcinoma

6

O. W. Hakenberg   K. Rüdiger   U. W. F. Wetterauer
H. Sommerkamp

Introduction

Cervical carcinoma occurs with equal frequency in all age groups above 25 years and remains the third most common malignancy in women, despite an overall declining incidence in many European countries. Whereas an increase in the incidence of cervical adenocarcinoma has been observed, the incidence of the more common squamous cell carcinoma, which accounts for more than 90% of cervical carcinomas, seems to be slowly declining.[1]

Radiotherapy remains one of the main therapeutic choices, with an efficacy similar to that of surgical treatment.[2] Staging of cervical carcinoma (Table 6.1), according to the classification of the International Federation

Stage	Description	Stage	Description
I	Cervical	IA	Less than 1 cm
		IB	1–1.5 cm
		IC	Large endometrial
II	Infiltrating	IIA	Upper vaginal
		IIB	Parametrial
III	Reaching lower vagina or pelvic wall		
IV	Bladder or enteric involvement		

Table 6.1. Classification of cervical carcinoma according to the International Federation of Gynecology and Obstetrics (FIGO) guidelines

of Gynecology and Obstetrics (FIGO), is based on pre-treatment clinical evaluation. Treatment consists of hysterectomy at stage IA, radical hysterectomy (Wertheim's operation) at stage IB and radiotherapy alone for all other stages. If the disease is more extensive than preoperative evaluation suggested, adjuvant postoperative radiotherapy is often employed. Alternatively, cervical carcinoma of all stages can be treated successfully by radiotherapy alone.

Usually, combined radiotherapy is used, with external beam irradiation plus intracavitary insertion of radioactive material. The radiotherapy regimen employed is dependent on several factors such as local extent of tumour, lymph node involvement and anatomical considerations. Standard regimens consist of intracavitary brachytherapy with caesium, cobalt or iridium in up to three applications of 15 Gy each for the genital target organs plus percutaneous 15×15 or 15×18 cm field irradiation with 25 MV photon radiation in fractionated doses for the parametrial regions as a supplementation. Total radiation doses of up to 50 Gy for the lateral pelvic wall and up to 70 Gy to the bladder are thus achieved.[3]

Cervical carcinoma itself is not particularly radiosensitive. Large radiation doses are therefore administered, because the radiation tolerance of the vagina and cervix is fairly high, and good cure rates can be achieved. However, the more radiosensitive adjacent organs in the pelvis, small bowel and rectum, as well as the urinary bladder and ureters, receive radiation doses that can well exceed their radiation tolerance. This can result in immediate side effects as well as permanent radiation damage, which may become apparent only after long lag periods.

There is some controversy concerning the frequency of urinary tract complications following radiotherapy for cervical carcinoma. In most series, only severe complications are counted, thereby somewhat underestimating total morbidity. Although many complications of radiotherapy appear relatively soon after completion of the treatment course, there is, however, evidence that late complications increase in frequency even 5 years after radiotherapy.[3] Although radiotherapy achieves relatively good rates of cure of the primary disease, it can (and not infrequently does) lead to late complications which, in themselves, can severely reduce the patient's quality of life or be life threatening.

This chapter reports on 16 patients with cervical carcinoma who had severe urinary tract complications from radiotherapy.

Patients and methods

A total of 16 patients with severe radiation complications, who were referred to the authors' unit during the last 2 years, were evaluated. These women had all received combined radiotherapy for stage IB or IIA cervical carcinoma (FIGO). The average age of the patients at presentation was 37.7 years, the average radiation dose had been 65 Gy and the mean latency time since radiotherapy was 1.8 years, with a range of 3 months to 22 years (Table 6.2). Of the 16 patients, 12 had undergone previous hysterectomy.

Half of the patients had been subjectively asymptomatic and had been referred by gynaecologists or general practitioners because of elevated serum creatinine levels or detection of renal obstruction on routine

Presenting symptom	Findings	Definitive treatment	Outcome
8 subjectively asymptomatic†	16 ureteral stenoses (4 bilateral)	For ureteral stenosis:	4 died
4 incontinent	7 fistulae	2 internal ureterotomies	1 lost to follow-up
4 with flank pain	12 reduced bladder compliance	2 ureteroneocystostomies	3 permanent nephrostomies
	6 with residual volume	5 double-J stents	4 urinary diversions
		2 ileal conduits	4 symptom-free after treatment
		For fistulae:	
		3 percutaneous nephrostomies	
		2 urinary diversions	

Table 6.2. Details of 16 patients* who presented to the authors' unit in 1992–93 with urological complications after radiotherapy for cervical carcinoma stage IB/IIA.
*Mean age, 37.7 years; mean radiation dose, 65 Gy; mean latency time, 1.8 years.
†Referral was for renal obstruction or elevated serum creatinine level.

ultrasound examination. The other patients were symptomatic, with frequency and pain on micturition, or symptoms of urinary fistulae.

All patients were evaluated by physical examination, urine culture, serum creatinine and electrolytes, ultrasound, residual urine and voiding function, intravenous pyelography, micturition cystograms and cystoscopy; some patients received retrograde pyelography, if necessary. In cases of renal obstruction, isotope nephrograms were performed. All patients were also re-evaluated by gynaecological consultation for recurrence of cervical carcinoma.

All patients had some degree of ureteral stenosis, most commonly distal ureteral stenosis (Fig. 6.1). Urinary tract fistulae were seen in seven patients: two of these fistulae were vesicovaginal, two vesico-intestinal (Fig. 6.2), two uretero-intestinal (Fig. 6.3) and one uretero-arterial. Fourteen patients had evidence of some degree of radiation cystitis with reduced bladder compliance, and 12 had disturbed bladder motility.

Treatment for the initial management of obstructive ureteral stenoses

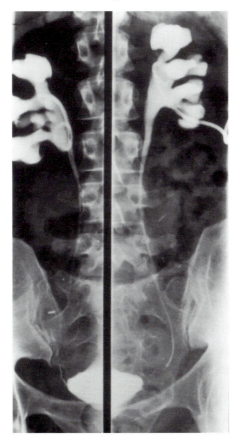

Figure 6.1. Bilateral distal ureteral stenoses in a 38-year-old patient following radiotherapy for cervical carcinoma. Bilateral percutaneous nephrostomies were inserted.

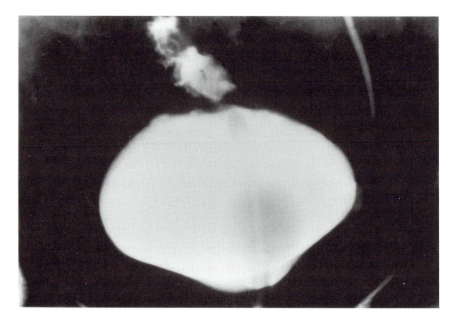

Figure 6.2. Vesico-intestinal fistula in a 57-year-old patient 15 years after radiotherapy for cervical carcinoma. Note also the distal ureteral stenosis on the left side.

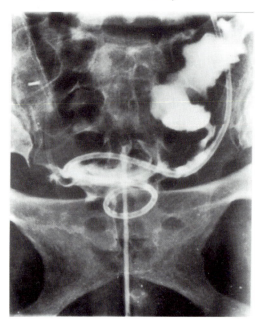

Figure 6.3. Uretero-intestinal fistula in a 42-year-old patient 3 years after radiotherapy for cervical carcinoma. Bilateral antegrade ureteral splinting was performed.

consisted of insertion of ureteral stents whenever possible; otherwise, percutaneous nephrostomies were inserted, if the affected kidney was still functioning according to isotope nephrograms or if infection of the obstructed kidney was present. In all cases of ureteral fistula, percutaneous nephrostomies or transurethral catheters were inserted for immediate management.

For definitive treatment after exclusion of tumour recurrence, urinary diversion by conduit or ureterocutaneostomy was performed in two patients with fistulae and in two with ureteral stenoses. Two patients with ureteral stenosis underwent ureteroneocystostomy; three patients remain with permanent ureteral stents (double-J stents).

Four patients eventually died. One patient with a left ureteric fistula to the common iliac artery died from acute bleeding after unsuccessful attempts at inserting a vascular stent; another patient with bilateral ureteral stenoses died from septicaemia. Two other patients were found to have tumour recurrence and died from disease progression. Only four of the 12 surviving patients are completely asymptomatic after urological treatment of their urinary tract complications from radiotherapy; four patients remain with urinary diversion and the consequent reduction in quality of life; three other patients have to undergo changing of double-J stents at regular intervals.

Discussion

It is well known that radiation damage to normal tissues is dependent on the organs involved, the dose of irradiation, fractionation and the volume treated. The assessment of the effectiveness of a treatment modality requires evaluation not only of the degree and probability of cure or tumour control but also of the likelihood and severity of morbidity induced by the treatment. Radiotherapy as a therapeutic modality for cervical carcinoma has been established as an effective treatment since the 1940s and has been widely used since. A variety of different treatment strategies and regimens exist, so that treatment results are often not directly comparable, but on the whole they do not differ a great deal. In most institutions, radiotherapy is used in combination with surgical treatment for early stages of invasive cervical carcinoma, either pre- or postoperatively, or both. Radiotherapy as the only treatment for cervical carcinoma is also highly effective,[4] with 5-year survival rates of 87% for stage IA, 73% for stage IIA and 68% for stage IIB. Similar results are reported by other authors.[5,6]

Because of the variations in treatment strategies and radiation modalities, the incidence of radiotherapy-induced morbidity and complications is not directly comparable and hence not entirely predictable. Moreover, the pretreatment staging according to the FIGO classification is not completely reliable, and has been shown to correspond to histological staging in only 60–70% of cases;[7,8] histological staging is, of course, achieved only in patients subjected to an operation. Histological evidence of pretreatment understaging usually leads to postoperative radiotherapy; thus, many patients receive radiotherapy after hysterectomy. In advanced stages of cervical carcinoma (stages IIB–IV) radiotherapy is the only treatment modality, with poorer survival rates.

The decreasing incidence of cervical squamous cell carcinoma has led to a relative increase in the number of older patients who, at the time of diagnosis of cervical carcinoma, have concomitant diseases and are generally more prone to develop early complications of any treatment. On the other hand, cytological screening for cervical carcinoma has also led to an increase in the diagnosis of early stages of the disease and a relative increase in the number of young patients treated. With the high cure rates achieved in the early disease stages of cervical carcinoma, late complications of treatment gain more importance for the long-term quality of life of these relatively young patients.

The absolute doses administered with standard radiotherapy add up to 75 Gy in the region of the urinary bladder base, and reach 45 Gy at the pelvic walls, with an expected incidence of severe radiation reactions of 5%, and of up to 30% if this dosage level is exceeded.[9] The degree and severity of radiation effects in the genitourinary tract are usually divided into early and late reactions. Clinical classifications for the assessment of radiation sequelae and injuries have been suggested;[10] however, exact classification seems difficult because of the overlap in clinical symptoms often observed.

That the urinary tract organs receive a certain radiation dose with radiotherapy of cervical carcinoma is inevitable and some degree of reaction will necessarily occur. Radiation will always directly damage tissue, which is the intended effect concerning the malignant target tissue. Acute tissue oedema, reactive hyperperfusion, cell death and necrosis will also occur to some degree in adjacent non-target tissues and account for early radiation reactions in the urinary tract. The pathological basis of long-term radiation injury seems to be closely related to vascular damage. Endothelial proliferations and capillary occlusion, arteriolar narrowing and intimal fibrosis occur after tissue radiation.[11] Vascular rarefications as a common change in major and minor pelvic vessels following radiotherapy have been documented in a series of 150 patients.[12]

The early morphological changes seen on cystoscopy are mucosal erythema, bullous oedema and telangiectasia. Telangiectasia is a sign of vascular damage with loss of vascular contractility and capillary atrophy, leading to reduced mucosal perfusion. This will often be asymptomatic, but may give rise to haematuria after sudden increases in intravesical pressure. Bullous oedema is a non-specific mucosal reaction also indicating impaired mucosal perfusion, and patchy erythema is also a common mucosal radiation reaction. Higher degrees of radiation reactions are mucosal ulcerations, with vascular erosions leading to gross haematuria and, if severe, to an ulcerative cystitis, often with bacterial superinfection, which can lead to deep ulceration and fistula formation as a late consequence. These early changes can occur during radiotherapy and can persist for weeks; there is great intra-individual variation and, although some degree of mucosal reaction can usually be seen on cystoscopy, they are mostly asymptomatic or cause only mild and transient symptoms of bladder irritation. However, severe early reactions may also cause severe irritative symptoms with frequency and pain; this clinical entity is usually called radiogenic cystitis, although secondary bacterial superinfections can occur. These changes are subject to repair mechanisms. However, even in asymptomatic patients, evidence of some degree of mucosal damage commonly persists and can be seen on cystoscopy.

Late radiation reactions in the bladder are end stages of these early reactions, in which a high degree of epithelial and muscular damage has occurred with inadequate repair. Secondary bacterial infections occur commonly and lead to further damage. If the destructive process reaches the whole bladder wall, fistulae will eventually form. Reduced vascular function and muscular atrophy due to radiation effects will lead to bladder shrinkage.

The reported incidence of radiation complications differs widely. The resulting controversy depends partly on the definition of radiation complications and their assessment and grading, and also on the intensity of radiotherapy as well as patient selection. Perez et al.[3] report an incidence of 5% of grade 2 and 3 urinary tract complications in a series of 811 patients with cervical carcinoma of all stages (including IA) treated by radiotherapy alone. They list chronic cystitis, ureteral stricture and incontinence under grade 2 complications, and chronic cystitis, bladder ulceration, fistulae and ureteral strictures as grade 3 complications. They do not report on the nature and frequency of grade 1 complications, and report a further incidence of 7% of grade 2 and 3 gastrointestinal complications and 6% of other grade 2 and 3 complications, adding up to a total of 18% of grades 2 and 3 complications. Grade 2 complications in their classification were those with 'major symptoms, repeated occurrence, often requiring hospitalization for non-surgical management' and grade 3 complications those which 'required major surgery for correction or were life threatening'. Five-year survival rates were high, with 87% for stage IB, 73% for stage IIA and 68% for stage IIB.

Koehler and Forberg[13] reported a lower incidence of 6% of late complications requiring therapeutic intervention in patients treated with radiotherapy for endometrial carcinoma; however, cumulative survival rates in this group were much lower, with 69% for stage IA, 64% for stage IB and 41% for stage II, indicating less intensive and less effective radiotherapy.

Staehler et al.,[14] looking at urological complications of all degrees in patients with endometrial carcinomas, found much higher incidences of pathological findings after radiotherapy; they reported 55.9% urological complications, most commonly in the bladder (55.2%), followed by the kidneys (21.6%) and the ureter (7.5%).

Pedersen et al.,[15] in a series of 442 patients with cervical carcinoma stages IIB to IV, concluded that the commonly practised reporting of radiotherapy complications, whereby the maximal damage only is counted for each patient, underestimates radiation morbidity. They used a system of successive morbidity scoring as a measure to estimate the burden of complications, and reported 27% of early complications and 10% of late complications for the urinary bladder. They also found that the frequency of late morbidity did not correlate with FIGO stage, whereas the successive morbidity scoring did; they concluded that this points to the importance of latency in reporting radiotherapeutic morbidity, i.e. patients with more advanced stages of their cervical carcinoma with poorer prognosis will have fewer late radiotherapy complications reported than patients with good disease control and long survival after radiotherapy.

Leonhardt and Ostry,[16] in an old series of 630 patients who were all free of tumour recurrence 6 months after radiotherapy for cervical carcinoma, found radiation-related changes of the urinary tract in 52.2% of cases, also evaluating all urinary tract pathology. The most common finding was clinical evidence of bladder irritability (23.6%), followed by urinary tract infection with 10.6%. Severe changes were less common: these included non-functioning kidney (1.6%), renal failure (0.3%), fistulae (0.8%) and ureteral stricture (0.3%). However, evidence of hydronephrosis was seen in 7.3% and bladder ulceration in 3.6%. This series, where the patients were evaluated by clinical evaluation, urine culture and intravenous pyelography, also illustrates that radiation effects on the urinary tract are more common, if changes of all degrees are evaluated.

The radiation tolerance of the urinary organs is not precisely known, although approximate values can be estimated. For the kidneys, a radiation dose of 10 Gy may cause damage and doses of 20 Gy probably will do so, resulting in glomerular and tubular injury with consecutive fibrosis.[12] For the ureter and the urinary bladder, estimated radiation tolerance values are given as 60–70 Gy. These radiation doses should normally not be exceeded. However, especially with intracavitary radiotherapy, higher doses will often be administered to parts of the bladder or segments of the ureter, since individual anatomical variations very often cause an eccentric, asymmetric position of the intracavitary radium load in the pelvis. It seems inevitable that the combination of percutaneous and intracavitary radiation will often lead to excessive local radiation doses to some portions of the lower urinary tract, owing to this common anatomical asymmetry.

It must be assumed that not all radiation complications become clinically manifest to their full extent. Earlier reports on autopsy material from the 1960s gave an incidence of 9–19% of ureteral stenoses after radiotherapy for cervical carcinoma,[17,18] and found the consequences of ureteral stenosis to be the second most common cause of death (next to tumour recurrence) in these patients.[16,19]

Many patients with cervical carcinoma already have disturbed ureteral function before therapy.[19] However, in 1919 cervical carcinoma patients with normal intravenous pyelograms and isotope nephrograms before radiotherapy, Breit[12] found evidence of functional distal ureteral obstruction in 30% soon after termination of radiotherapy, 87% of which returned to normal several months later. He reported an incidence of late severe ureteral stenoses of 1.8% and permanent manifest evidence of distal functional ureteral obstruction of 9–10%.

Although radiation injuries to the pelvic non-target organs have thus been described, the period of risk for their development and manifestation is not well defined.[3,8,10] The time course of the appearance of radiation damage in the urinary tract is variable. The latest manifestations in the present authors' patient group was 22 years; Zoubek et al.[20] reported a case of 39 years, while Pedersen et al.,[15] in their 10-year retrospective analysis, found almost all complications within 3–4 years after radiotherapy. Kan and Afanas[21] reported a mean interval of 5.6 years after pelvic radiotherapy for the manifestation of ureteral strictures. However, it seems clear from the cases presented that radiation damage can become apparent years— sometimes decades—after successful radiotherapy for cervical carcinoma. These late manifestations may well be related to other intercurrent illnesses, such as atherosclerosis or diabetes mellitus, which later appear in patients with long-term survival after radiotherapy and may further damage urinary tract tissue already functionally impaired by radiation effects. Radiation complications are, therefore, likely to increase with time. Staehler et al.[14] found a 68.9% higher incidence of pathological urological findings in patients 5 years after radiotherapy compared with 1 year after radiotherapy.

Even without the clinical manifestation of radiation injuries, changes in the urinary bladder occur and can be of functional consequence. Kümper[22] found some degree of reduced bladder compliance, which was not radiation-dose dependent, in most patients with urodynamic evaluation even 5 years after radiotherapy. In animal experiments with higher radiation doses, a clear dose-dependent impairment of bladder function could be established.[23] This loss of normal storage function with an increase in intravesical pressure, which is volume related, is generally associated with uncomfortable and irritative bladder symptoms and can result in urinary incontinence and/or ureteral obstruction. Since low-pressure accommodation of the urine volume is compromised with a loss of adequate reservoir function of the bladder, operative repair of vesicovaginal fistulae may fail in these cases.[20]

Risk factors for the development of radiation injuries are poorly defined. From the above, it seems clear that there is a high degree of intra-individual patient variability and the occurrence and degree of radiation reactions cannot be predicted accurately for the individual patient. There is a reported higher incidence of vascular complications of radiotherapy for cervical carcinoma in smokers.[24] There is also a definitely increased risk in patients who previously underwent pelvic surgery, which is often the case in cervical carcinoma patients.

Urinary tract infections are a further risk factor. Kümper[25] found bacteriuria in 50% of cervical carcinoma patients during radiotherapy; half of these were asymptomatic. The bacterial spectrum did not differ from that of ordinary urinary tract infections. The risk of urinary tract contamination in cervical carcinoma patients is increased, owing to repeated instrumenta-tion of the lower urinary and genital tract before and during radiotherapy. Bialas et al.,[26] in a prospective study in patients receiving pelvic radiotherapy, found 17% of urinary tract infections before, and a further 17% during, radiotherapy.

The most common pathological finding in the present authors' patient group was distal ureteral obstruction, which was often asymptomatic to the patient and endangered renal function. Kan and Afanas[21] reported on 58 cases of ureteral obstruction in patients following pelvic radiotherapy for uterine or bladder cancer, and found short distal ureteral strictures in 69% and long strictures in 31%. In the present authors' opinion, it therefore seems necessary to screen regularly all patients, after radiotherapy for cervical carcinoma, for the often asymptomatic development of renal obstruction due to ureteral stenosis, in order to prevent renal damage by early intervention. Whether early or even prophylactic insertion of ureteral double-J stents will prevent further ureteral stricture formation is not known.

For practical clinical considerations, the authors suggest that radiation sequelae should be classified into early and late complications of different degrees (Table 6.3). Early radiation complications become apparent mainly with symptoms related to the urinary bladder, and are often of a transient nature; however, symptoms may be severe, but will not persist with the same intensity. Morphological changes can be seen on cystoscopy, but these will be subject to repair mechanisms, although often incompletely.

Early reactions:
  mild: irritative bladder symptoms
    (mucosal oedema/erythema)
  moderate: marked bladder irritation, haematuria
    (marked mucosal bullous oedema/erythema)
  severe: severe bladder irritation, painful haematuria
    (severe mucosal oedema/erythema/ulcerations)

Late reactions:
  mild: persisting bladder irritation, reduced compliance, ureteral stenosis without
    obstruction
    (patchy mucosal atrophy/telangiectasia)
  moderate: severe persisting bladder irritation, highly reduced bladder compliance,
    ureteral stenosis with obstruction requiring intervention
    (patchy mucosal atrophy/telangiectasia)
  severe: severe bladder shrinkage, complete ureteral obstruction, vesical or ureteral
    fistulae requiring intervention/repair
    (severe patchy mucosal atrophy/ulcerations)

Table 6.3. Suggested classification of radiation reactions and sequelae in the urinary tract*
*The presence of bacterial urinary tract infection does not exclude radiation reactions.

Concomitant urinary tract infections are common, and will increase the severity of symptoms as well as the risk of further damage; therefore, bacterial urinary tract infection does not necessarily exclude symptoms from being related to previous radiotherapy, but has to be looked for and treated. Late complications are characterized by a variable latency period and by more permanent symptoms of constant severity, and will often require endo-urological or surgical procedures.

Whereas early radiation complications require the exclusion of urinary tract infection and symptomatic treatment only, evaluation of late radiation complications in the genitourinary tract needs a complete urological diagnostic work-up in order to assess the severity of the complication and to determine the need for adequate therapy. This necessitates the exclusion of bacterial infection; ultrasound and intravenous pyelography to detect evidence of ureteral stenosis and renal obstruction; evaluation of renal function by serum creatinine measurement and isotope nephrogram, if renal obstruction has been present for an unknown or longer period; cystoscopy for evaluation of bladder mucosal morphology and/or evaluation and localization of fistulae, in combination with retrograde ureteropyelography if ureteral stenosis is suspected; voiding cystography for voiding function and, again, fistula localization; as well as urinary flow measurement, residual volume determination and urodynamic evaluation for assessment of bladder function.

A full evaluation will reveal the degree and nature of urinary tract damage. Management will depend on the degree of damage and its functional consequences. Immediate management to relieve obstruction or incontinence due to fistulae will require insertion of ureteral stents, percutaneous nephrostomy or catheter drainage of the bladder; concomitant urinary tract infection must be treated. Severe, chronically reduced bladder compliance with incapacitating symptoms may need bladder augmentation; fistulae will require surgical closure; severe and obstructing ureteral stenoses may need ureteral reimplantation or urinary diversion, if severe bladder damage is present as well, which is often the case. A uretero-arterial fistula, which developed in one of the authors' cases, is a rare complication, of which fewer than 20 cases have been described.[27] The prognosis is poor, as surgical intervention with vascular repair will be difficult. In the case in question, the patient was also suspected to have tumour recurrence; therefore, only palliative measures were tried.

In summary, the frequency of radiation damage to urinary tract organs in radiotherapy of cervical carcinoma is often underestimated, owing to the assessment of severe damage only. With effective cure from the underlying life-threatening disease, some degree of radiation-induced damage to non-target tissues is inevitable and has to be accepted. Manifest radiation damage is largely related to vascular damage; thus, all factors further impairing vascular perfusion—such as previous pelvic surgery, atherosclerosis, diabetes mellitus, or a history of smoking—will increase the individual risk for the development of severe radiation sequelae. Regarding surgery for cervical carcinoma, the risk is the same, whether radiotherapy is administered before or after surgery, or both.[28] Urinary tract infection, which is common in cervical carcinoma patients during therapy, is a further definite risk factor that has to be looked for and treated.

The better the individual survival after radiotherapy, the more likely the patient will be to develop late sequelae of radiotherapy, since the later development of intercurrent illnesses that further impair perfusion of the pelvic organs will increase the risk of the late development of radiation-related damage.

The increase in the number of young women with early stages of cervical carcinoma, due to successful screening methods, and their long-term survival, due to effective treatment, makes awareness of the risk and screening for late radiotherapy complications particularly important. Occult ureteral stenoses are a common finding in this group of patients, as the authors' patient group demonstrates, and should be looked for before permanent renal damage has occurred.

References

1. Leminen A, Paavonen J, Forss M et al. Adenocarcinoma of the uterine cervix. Cancer 1990; 65: 53–59

2. Morley G W, Seski J C. Radical pelvic surgery versus radiation therapy for stage I carcinoma of the cervix (exclusive of microinvasion). Am J Obstet Gynecol 1976; 123: 785–792

3. Perez C A, Breaux S, Bedwinek J M et al. Radiation therapy alone in the treatment of carcinoma of the uterine cervix. II. Analysis of complications. Cancer 1984; 54: 235–246

4. Perez C A, Breaux S, Madoc-Jones H et al. Radiation therapy alone in the treatment of carcinoma of the uterine cervix. I. Analysis of tumour recurrence. Cancer 1983; 51: 1393–1402

5. Pettersson F. Behandlungsergebnisse des Zervixkarzinoms. Erkenntnisse aus dem FIGO-Jahresbericht. In: Teufel G, Pfleiderer A, Ladner H A (eds) Therapie des Zervixkarzinoms. Berlin: Springer-Verlag, 1990; 211–220

6. Boyce J, Fruchter R, Nicastri A et al. Prognostic factors in stage I carcinoma of the cervix. Gynecol Oncol 1981; 12: 154–158

7. Baltzer J. Die Bewertung prognostischer Kriterien bei Karzinomen des Uterus. Geburtshilfe Frauenheilkd 1981; 41: 663–667

8. Van Nagell J R, Roddick J W, Lowin D M. The staging of cervical cancer: inevitable discrepancies between staging and pathological findings. Am J Obstet Gynecol 1971; 110: 973–977

9. Kümper H J. Postaktinische Reaktionen des Harntraktes. In: Petri E (ed) Gynäkologische Urologie. Stuttgart: Thieme, 1983; 87–97

10. Kottmeier H L, Gray M J. Rectal and bladder injuries in relation to radiation dosage in carcinoma of the cervix. Am J Obstet Gynecol 1961; 81: 74–79

11. Zollinger H U. Handbuch der Allgemeinen Pathologie. Berlin: Springer-Verlag, 1978; 10: 234–236

12. Breit A. Vermeidbare und unvermeidbare Strahlenreaktionen bei der Behandlung des Kollumkarzinoms. In: Schmaehl D (ed) Prophylaxe und Therapie von Behandlungsfolgen bei Karzinomen der Frau. Stuttgart: Thieme, 1976; 26–30

13. Koehler U, Forberg J. Therapieregebnisse bei 718 Endometriumkarzinomen unter Beruecksichtigung klinischer und morphologischer Prognosefaktoren. Zentralbl Gynakol 1989; 111: 1033–1041

14. Staehler G, Leonhardt A, Knapp A, Wieland W. Urologic complications following radiotherapy of cancers of the corpus uteri. Geburtshilfe Frauenheilkd 1985; 45: 630–633

15. Pedersen D, Bentzen S, Overgaard J. Early and late radiotherapeutic morbidity in 442 consecutive patients with locally advanced carcinoma of the uterine cervix. Int J Radiat Oncol Biol Phys 1994; 29: 941–952

16. Leonhardt A, Ostry P. Behandlungsfolgen aus der Sicht einer Krebs-Nachsorgeklinik. In: Schmaehl D (ed) Prophylaxe und Therapie von Behandlungsfolgen bei Karzinomen der Frau. Stuttgart, Thieme, 1976; 14–22

17. Krichhoff H. Komplikationsreiche Veraenderungen am Harnsystem nach Strahlentherapie des Collumkarzinoms. Geburtshilfe Frauenheilkd 1960; 10: 34–39

18. Heller K L, Kaeser O. Todesursachen beim Collumkarzinom. Geburtshilfe Frauenheilkd 1966; 26: 155–164

19. Breit A. Harnabflußstörungen als Komplikation nach Radio-Therapie. Langenbecks Arch Chir 1969; 325: 644–651

20. Zoubek J, McGuire E J, Noll F, DeLancey J O. The late occurrence of urinary tract damage in patients successfully treated by radiotherapy for cervical carcinoma. J Urol 1989; 141: 1347–1349

21. Kan I, Afanas M B. Ureteral obstruction after radiotherapy in patients with cancer. Urol Nefrol 1989; 2: 31–34

22. Kümper H J. Zum funktionellen Verhalten der Harnblase bei der Therapie des Uteruskarzinoms mit ionisierenden Strahlen. Thesis, Munich, 1972

23. Michailov M C, Welscher U E, Kümper H J. Immediate contractile response of guinea-pig urinary bladder in situ to x-irradiation. Strahlentherapie 1974; 148: 409–414

24. Pettersson B, Swedenborg J. Localized arterial occlusion in patients treated with pelvic field irradiation for cancer. Soc Pelvic Surg 37th Annual Meet; Rome, 1987

25. Kümper H J. Infektionsbelastung der Harnblase während gynäkologischer Strahlentherapie. Munch Med Wochenschr 1971; 113: 1653–1654

26. Bialas I, Bessell E, Sokal M, Slack R. A prospective study of urinary tract infection during pelvic radiotherapy. Radiother Oncol 1989; 16: 305–309

27. Sparwasser C, Kugler A, Gilbert P et al. Bilateral ureteroiliac fistula coincident with radiotherapy and ureteral splint. Urologe A 1994; 33: 85–87
28. Hohenfellner R J. Die urologischen Komplikationen des Collum-Karzinoms. Berlin, Springer-Verlag, 1965

Surgical salvage of the postirradiation frozen pelvis

7

C. R. Chapple   R. T. Turner-Warwick

Introduction

Cancer is the major cause of death in women aged 35–54. Radiotherapy using a combination of local intracavity radiation and external beam therapy is used in combination with surgery for the treatment of many of the gynaecological malignancies. Although improved imaging, planning for radiotherapy and actual dose delivery have improved markedly in recent years, there always remains the potential risk of damage to 'normal' tissues in the pelvis at the time of irradiation for gynaecological cancer. Currently, serious sequelae from radiotherapy are uncommon in contemporary practice. Nevertheless, when they do occur they result in considerable morbidity for the patient, often with catastrophic effects on the patient's lifestyle, particularly as the patients are often relatively young.

Milder forms of radiation cystitis and proctitis and lesser degrees of vaginal damage usually resolve with either conservative management or local pharmacotherapeutic measures. The extent of more severe damage is often difficult to assess preoperatively because of the close anatomical juxtaposition of the lower urinary tract and the lower gastrointestinal tract to the vagina and uterus. In addition, there is often concern over the presence of residual neoplasia. Severe radiation-related problems within the pelvis therefore represent a significant surgical challenge.

In this chapter the authors review several cases that illustrate the surgical principles involved in the management of severe radiation-related injuries to the pelvic viscera. The authors first give a general appraisal of their personal approach to the management of urinary tract fistulae and the role of the omentum, before more specific comments on how to approach the patient with a significant radiation-induced injury to the pelvic viscera.

Urinary tract fistulae: the use of pedicle flaps and the role of omentum

Fistulous communications between the urinary tract and adjacent structures are a cause of great distress to the patient. Few patients are more anxious to be cured of their affliction, or are more grateful when this has been accomplished. The vast majority of such fistulae occur in women and result from gynaecological or obstetric trauma—most commonly urinary vaginal fistulae involving the bladder, ureter and rarely the urethra.

Vesico-intestinal communications usually occur as a complication of inflammatory or malignant bowel disease, with the exception of the relatively rare case of the radiation-damaged 'frozen pelvis' following treatment of gynaecological malignancy, which is the subject of the latter part of this review. Urethrorectal and urethrocutaneous fistulae are the only group that occur most commonly in men.

The subdivision of fistulae into 'simple' and 'complex' introduces further nomenclature. At first sight this might be considered to complicate matters unnecessarily; however, it serves a useful purpose in defining the appropriate surgical repair. Simple fistulae can usually be resolved by a simple closure in layers. More complex cases with associated tissue devascularization, previous failed surgical repair attempts or irradiation, extensive tissue loss, or persistence of a focus of infection or malignancy may require the use of adjunctive procedures such as omental interposition. Almost all fistulae, whether traumatic, surgical, inflammatory, neoplastic or radiation induced, are amenable to surgical repair.

Definition of the precise anatomical abnormality is necessary before taking a decision on the appropriate management of a fistula. The combined use of imaging modalities and a careful examination under anaesthetic are an essential preliminary in the repair of fistulae, since in many cases more than one structure (for example both the bladder and the ureter) is involved in the fistula. In addition, the demonstration of associated functional abnormalities and the presence of malignant disease are all important contributory factors that need to be considered and investigated before undertaking reparative surgery.

The basic surgical option for the repair of a vesical fistula lies between a vaginal-approach procedure and an abdominal-approach procedure. Many surgeons have an instinctive personal preference for one or other of these, but this is not as it should be. Although many simple vesicovaginal fistulae can be closed by a vaginal repair procedure, the access that this provides is relatively restricted and any significant incidence of failure after this suggests underusage of the abdominal approach. Similarly, a significant incidence of failure after a simple abdominal-approach layer closure can be resolved by a formal omental-interposition procedure, because, in the absence of active tumour or infection, this procedure should be almost invariably successful. Thus the most reliable fistula-closure procedure must be the 'three option' (vaginal–abdominal–omental) progression approach procedure and almost the only indication for urinary diversion after a fistula operation is urinary incontinence due to irremediable sphincter damage.

Conservative management

What are the indications for surgery versus conservative treatment?

In the case of ureteric fistulae, if a stent can be passed easily, then, after passage of the stent, a conservative approach is reasonable and a number of these fistulae will heal. Few vesicovaginal fistulae, close spontaneously. Marshall reported only one case in a series of 92 patients.[1]

A number of adjuvant measures have been used in addition to drainage: (a) local or systemic oestrogen therapy;[2] (b) antibiotic prophylaxis;[3] (c) cystoscopic fulguration of the fistula,[4] and (d) corticosteroid therapy.[5] None of these have been particularly successful and it must be concluded that the great majority of vesicovaginal fistulae fail to heal if treated conservatively. Such fistulae should be considered to be a urological emergency, particularly as there may be associated medicolegal implications. The only exceptions to this are those that occur immediately post partum—where other factors, such as uterine involution, need to be taken into account.

Treatment of urethral fistulae, on the other hand, should hardly ever be rushed into, because of the associated damage to the intrinsic urethral sphincter mechanism. In many of these cases, attention to sphincteric function is necessary by the use of an appropriate repair technique such as sphincteroplasty.

Timing of surgery

It is difficult to generalize about the appropriate timing of surgical intervention for every case, as this will depend upon the systemic and local factors influencing the healing potential of the local tissues in the individual case. It is almost invariably possible to resolve ureteric and vesical fistulae by early exploration within the first 2 weeks, before the process of inflammation and repair render surgery difficult. The majority of evidence suggests that if this window of opportunity is missed it is wise to defer surgery for at least 3 months,[1,6] as it would be inapprophriate to carry out a surgical procedure that would potentially be rendered more complex and extensive and where morbidity is likely to be higher. In more complex fistulae, where tissue healing is dependent on the interposition of a pedicled flap of vascularized tissue such as omentum, this timing is less critical to healing of the fistula, but surgery carried out at an inappropriate time may be rendered far more difficult. Although some workers have advocated repair between 3 and 12 weeks,[7,8] it must be remembered that these cases were all repaired by the use of interposed flaps of peritoneum or omentum. It is salutary that in a reported series of 11 'early' repairs of vesicovaginal fistula, 10 cases were successfully operated on before 3 weeks had elapsed after injury; in the remaining case, a repair by simple layer closure at 35 days broke down on the fifth postoperative day.[9]

Choice of approach

The ensuing discussion refers to vesicovaginal fistulae predominantly, but similar concepts are equally vital in determining the appropriate approach to other urinary tract fistulae. The decision as to the best surgical approach for an individual case will, of course, be considerably biased by an individual surgeon's preference and training. It will also depend upon the aetiology, position and size of the vesical fistula and the concurrence of associated ureteric or urethral damage. Adequate surgical access to the fistula itself, to allow associated procedures such as urethral repair, ureteric reimplantation or the interposition of pedicle flaps, is essential to a successful repair. These requirements should be the most important factor in determining the surgical approach.

A perineal approach provides limited access but avoids the morbidity associated with any abdominal procedure. It is ideally suited to closure of the low simple fistula and can be combined with the use of an interposed pedicled flap of labial/scrotal tissue or gracilis muscle, for more complex fistulae. The abdominal approach is more invasive for the patient but is indicated for the repair of high or complex fistulae, and lends itself to the concomitant interposition of a pedicled omental flap in the repair. The most logical approach is to have available the expertise to use all the available procedures as most appropriate,[10,11] preparing the patient for a synchronous perineo-abdominal procedure at the outset of an operation and thereby facilitating the progression of one to the other as necessary.[6]

Repair technique

The plethora of case reports and techniques described in the literature bear witness not only to the variation in the success of the different surgical methods in the hands of individual surgeons but also to the diversity of different procedures that are available. Any surgical repair will succeed, provided that it removes any predisposing aetiological cause for a fistula and reconstitutes a defect by the approximation of clean, well-vascularized tissue. These criteria are easily achieved in simple fistulae by the trimming and tension-free approximation of adjacent wound edges. In more complex cases, where the fistulous defect is large or where fibrosis resulting from infection, surgery or irradiation compromises tissue healing, the interposition of a pedicled flap of well-vascularized tissue markedly increases the chances of a successful repair. In these cases it must be remembered that, if the tension-free apposition of an epithelial defect is not possible, the migration of epithelial cells will occur over an interposed vascularized pedicled flap; it is, therefore, perfectly acceptable to leave defects, provided that they are adequately covered by the flap.

Vaginal repair of the complex fistula

Simple fistulae can often be closed by the use of a direct closure of the tissue defect. In some cases the local vaginal tissues are damaged to the extent that a simple layered closure of the vagina is felt to be potentially precarious; such a situation may result from tissue loss or tissue fibrosis produced by infection or previous surgery. In this situation it is necessary to augment the operation by the interposition of a vascularized flap between the two layers of the repair, filling dead space and bringing in a much-needed blood and lymphatic supply. Many of these fistulae can be repaired using a vaginal procedure.

A number of techniques have been described for the mobilization and deployment of adjacent soft tissue structures: these include transposition of the medial fibres of the levator ani,[12] use of a gracilis muscle flap,[13–15] or a gracilis myocutaneous flap[16] and the use of a pedicle flap of vulval fat and bulbocavernosus muscle.[17] Although the use of procedures utilizing the gracilis is invaluable for the repair of extensive defects, the majority of cases can be satisfactorily resolved by the use of a Martius flap;[17] this procedure is therefore described in detail here.

A vertical incision is made in either labium majus, allowing a posteriorly based pedicled vascularized flap of labial tissue to be raised. The size of the flap is determined by the size of the fistula and can be increased by anterior extension of the incision into the mons. The flap is mobilized, taking care not to damage the blood supply from the inferior haemorrhoidal vessels that enter anteriorly. Next, a tunnel is made beneath a vulval skin bridge to the site of fistula closure. The labial flap is secured in position as part of the final layer closure.

A problem encountered occasionally is that of a urethrovaginal fistula. The majority of those patients with a distal urethrovaginal fistula are continent and asymptomatic, provided that the bladder neck mechanism is competent.[18] Vaginal repair of such a fistula is easily carried out. If there is an associated urethral mucosal defect, it can be replaced by a suitable flap of adjacent vaginal mucosa supported by a Martius flap. Alternatively, a modification of the Martius procedure can be used, whereby the urethral repair is facilitated by a suitably positioned skin island left on the labial pedicle.[19] If the fistula is more proximal and a more extensive repair of urethra is likely to be necessary, or if it is associated with a vesicovaginal fistula, then a combined transvesical and abdominal approach is preferable.

Abdominal repair of urinary tract fistulae

Exposure

The patient is placed in the same position as that outlined above for the vaginal approach. A midline incision should always be used for the abdominal approach to a fistula repair, because it is often necessary to extend this up to the xiphisternum to provide the necessary access for mobilization of a short omentum. A more cosmetic result can be achieved—particularly in those patients who have recently undergone a gynaecological procedure via a Pfannenstiel incision—by reopening the transverse skin incision and then making a vertical incision through the abdominal wall musculature, with an additional upper midline incision to aid omental mobilization if this proves to be necessary.

Dissection

A combined transperitoneal–transvesical approach to a vesicovaginal fistula is to be preferred over the conventional anterior transvesical approach[20] first described by Trendelenburg in 1890 and subsequently modified.[21] This is important, as it allows good access to the area of the fistula and facilitates separation of the bladder from the vagina, with the formation of an abdominoperineal tunnel that provides a good extravesical exposure of the terminal ureters.[22] An initial incision is made into the vesicovaginal peritoneal fold and the posterior wall of the bladder is opened in the midline down to the fistula (Fig. 7.1a). Separation of the vaginal vault from the bladder is facilitated by an orientating finger placed within the vagina. A three-finger-breadth abdominoperineal tunnel is completed in the plane between bladder and vagina; it is important to create a suitable 'space' to allow the adequate tension-free redeployment of a suitable bulk of omentum. In difficult cases and, in particular, in those

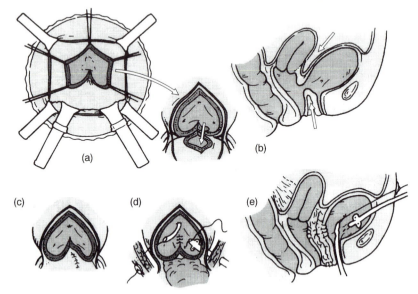

Figure 7.1. (a) Abdominal exposure to a vesicovaginal fistula, showing the importance of good exposure using a ring retractor. The bladder is opened by a laterally curved posterior incision down to the fistula and the plane between bladder and vagina is opened up, taking care not to injure the ureters. (b) In difficult cases, an abdominoperineal tunnel is developed in this plane to receive the omentum. (c) The vaginal and bladder defect is closed. (d,e) The omentum is deployed and bladder closure is carried out. Both suprapubic and urethral catheters are used, to ensure adequate drainage.

where previous surgery has been attempted, the abdominal dissection can be combined with a subsequent perineal dissection to produce an abdominoperineal tunnel, thereby allowing linear deployment of the omentum along the whole length of the vagina[22] (Fig. 7.1b).

Closure

The vagina is closed with an absorbable 3/0 suture (Fig. 7.1c). Although many simple fistulae can be satisfactorily closed using this approach with a layer closure as described above, an additional advantage can be gained by the addition of an omental pedicled flap in the closure[23] (Fig. 7.1d,e), which is interposed in the abdominoperineal tunnel. The bladder is closed with a similar absorbable suture and adequate drainage ensured by the use of combined urethral and suprapubic drainage, the repair being wrapped in omentum. This surgical technique is applicable to a wide variety of fistulae and provides a virtually guaranteed closure of most fistulae.[24] At the end of the procedure a colposuspension may be carried out where necessary to reposition the proximal urethra and bladder neck, ensuring the optimal transmission of intra-abdominal pressure and thereby militating against the development of stress incontinence.[25]

The use of pedicled interposition flaps

The interposition of well-vascularized tissue such as omentum, as described above, brings in a good blood supply and fills dead space. This acts as an added safeguard of a successful result in simple fistulae, and it is essential to the closure of a complex fistula.

A number of techniques have been described in the literature: these include the use of peritoneal interposition,[26,27] first described by Bardescu in 1900, the use of island myocutaneous and fasciocutaneous flaps,[28,29] of bladder mucosa[30] and of omentum, which was first reported by Walters[23] in 1935 and subsequently developed by Kiricuta and Goldstein[31] and elaborated by Turner-Warwick et al.[32] in the last three decades. Omentum should be the first choice in all cases. This tissue serves the function within the abdomen of sealing off and localizing areas of infection. It is readily available and easy to mobilize, reaching down to the perineum in most cases; it has an excellent vascular and lymphatic supply and has sufficient bulk to fill dead space without producing marked fibrosis during healing—which might compromise lower urinary tract function and render subsequent surgery more difficult. In contrast, peritoneum, although being readily available, does not possess these other properties and is likely to have been involved in local pathology or included in the irradiated field. Bladder mucosal grafts can be used in a manner analogous to vaginal mucosa, but carry the same potential disadvantages as suggested for peritoneum. Other flap procedures are an important part of the armamentarium but require particular expertise.

The omentum should always be separated from its attachment to the transverse colon and mesocolon, as postoperative distension of the bowel may otherwise dislodge its attachment to the subsequent repair. The lower margin of the omental apron will reach the perineum without additional mobilization in 30% of cases (Fig. 7.2a). In the remaining cases, some degree of mobilization of the omentum by division of part of its vascular pedicle is necessary. Although Kiricuta originally mobilized the omentum on the left gastro-epiploic arch, this vessel usually becomes increasingly small towards its left extremity and the omental flap should be based on the right gastro-epiploic pedicle for a more reliable blood supply[32] (Fig. 7.3). In approximately 30% of cases, sufficient elongation is achieved by division of the left gastro-epiploic pedicle (Fig. 7.2b). In the remaining 40% of cases, full mobilization is required on the right gastro-epiploic vessel right over to its gastroduodenal origin to prevent undue traction on individual short gastric vessels, which might result in shearing and postoperative haemorrhage. Careful ligation of individual short gastric vessels is necessary, using an absorbable suture (Fig. 7.2c). The resultant slender vascular pedicle of this flap is protected by relocating it behind the mobilized descending colon. Mobilization of the omentum from the stomach tends to result in a mild ileus and it is therefore sensible to institute gastric suction for a few days postoperatively; the insertion of a gastrostomy tube is a humane alternative to a nasogastric tube—as the stomach is suitably exposed.

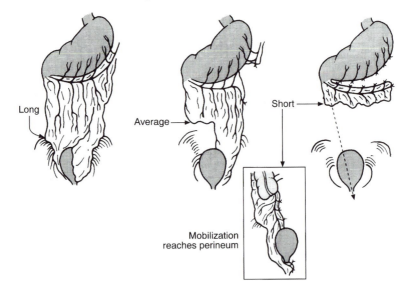

Figure. 7.2. (a) In approximately 30% of cases the omentum will reach the pelvis without mobilization. (b) In a further 30% of cases the omentum can be adequately lengthened by division of its lateral lieno-renal ligament attachments. (c) Full mobilization of the omentum on the right gastro-epiploic pedicle is necessary in the remaining 40% of patients. The omentum is led down into the pelvis along the right paracolic gutter behind the mobilized right colon (insert).

The repair of complex fistulae

In the authors' experience, the repair of complex urinary tract fistulae is mostly reliably resolved via the abdominoperineal approach, with omental interposition as described above.[24] Certain additional points are, however, worthy of comment.

If radiotherapy is implicated in the aetiology of the fistula, the wall of the bladder is usually rendered more rigid and inflexible than is normally the case. In this situation, a curved incision in the wall of the bladder is often preferable to one in the midline, as this facilitates subsequent bladder closure by the rotation of a broad-based bladder flap. In those patients with radiation-induced fibrosis and necrosis, the surgical procedure must be considered to consist of two separate stages. It is first necessary to *excise* all macroscopically abnormal tissue. If residual malignancy is suspected, this can be confirmed by frozen section, but, unless extensive, apart from biasing the surgeon towards a more radical excision, should not preclude a reconstructive procedure. The second stage of this operation involves a *functional restoration* of the integrity of the rectum, bladder and vagina, as far as this is feasible, filling the dead space within the (inevitably) ischaemic pelvis with omentum and/or a caecocolovaginoplasty.[25]

If there is an extensive defect, then it may not be possible to obtain satisfactory apposition of the edges of the bladder wall without comprom-

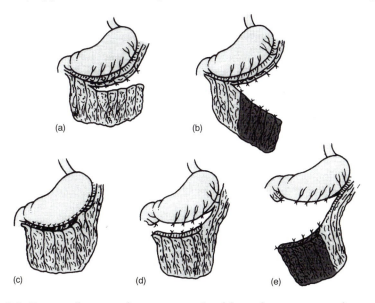

Figure. 7.3. Diagram illustrating the importance of mobilizing the omentum on the appropriate vascular arcade. In the situation illustrated in (a) it can be seen that the omentum has been erroneously mobilized distal to the gastro-epiploic arcade. The consequence will be ischaemic loss and consequently (b) necrosis of the mobilized omentum. (c) A typical case where the left gastro-epiploic arcade is incomplete. Incorrect technique for mobilization on the gastro-epiploic arcade (d) has resulted (e) in ischaemia of the mobilized omentum.

ising its functional capacity. Closure of the bladder defect can be carried out with the additional use of an augmentation cystoplasty. Alternatively, the bladder defect can be left and the omentum used to patch it—animal studies have clearly demonstrated that the defect is covered, within 2–3 weeks, by new transitional epithelium, with the subsequent formation of a new smooth muscle layer within the omentoplasty in continuity with the margins of the detrusor muscle at the edges of the defect.[33,34] Clinical experience over the last 25 years has confirmed the efficacy of this technique in the clinical setting.[32,35,36]

Lower urinary tract fistulae in men

Although the great majority of lower urinary tract fistulae occur in women, men occasionally develop a urethrocutaneous or recto-urethral fistula, usually resulting from trauma or inflammatory bowel disease. It is important to exclude malignancy as a cause of the fistula by preoperative investigations, particularly in those patients in whom the fistula complicates a previous abdominoperineal resection for adenocarcinoma of the rectum. A number of perineal approaches have been described and used successfully for the repair of these fistulae. However, in the authors' experience they can be most easily and reliably repaired using the abdominoperineal approach, with the formation of an abdominoperineal tunnel and omental interposition, as described above.[24]

Urethrocutaneous fistulae in women

The principles underlying urethral fistula repair are similar to those associated with the resolution of a vesicovaginal fistula. An additional potential factor to bear in mind is that urinary continence is entirely dependent upon the function of the intrinsic urethral sphincter musculature within the thickness of the urethral wall. A urethrovaginal fistula is invariably associated with a defect in the posterior section of the urethral sphincter mechanism. Repair of such an injury should, therefore, be combined with an appropriate repair of the urethral sphincter mechanism.[36]

Upper urinary tract fistulae

Surgical injuries to the ureter are most commonly located in its lower third. Not infrequently, an associated ureteric injury is distal, in conjunction with a vesical fistula. Injuries of the middle and upper third of the ureter are rare. Whenever possible, if the injury is detected at an early enough stage, a simple end-to-end spatulated overlap anastomotic repair should be used. After the first few postoperative days, local peri-ureteric tissue reaction may compromise such a repair, especially when the lesion is low in the pelvis. In these circumstances, a bladder-elongation psoas-hitch procedure is the best approach, in the authors' opinion.[37] An important feature of this procedure is an initial bladder-elongating hemicircumferential incision in the equatorial line of the bladder, because it is this that enables the dome of the bladder to be advanced upwards without tension. Repair of a ureteric fistula on any level can be very usefully supported by the adjacent deployment of omentum, which brings in a new vascular supply, thereby helping to seal any repair and maintain the suppleness of the repaired tissues by preventing direct peri-ureteric fibrosis.

The surgical approach to the irradiated pelvis

Although it is well recognized from the literature that radiation can have disastrous consequences, this is an uncommon complication and few centres have amassed significant experience of the surgical management of postirradiation pelvic injuries, with a few exceptions.[38,39] Other series in the literature comprise case reports,[40] but all reiterate the traditional approach to such injuries, which is the repair of simple fistulae, and urinary and faecal diversion in more complex cases.[41–43]

In a number of cases there is no doubt that the presence of extensive recurrent malignancy, coexistence of other medical pathology and, of course, patients' wishes, will militate against a radical surgical approach. Having stated this it must, however, be remembered that even when a severely radiation-damaged pelvis has been defunctioned, it can often be the site of recurrent infections and troublesome unpleasant discharge via the residual fistulae from the infected damaged pelvic cavity. In addition, the presence of malignant disease, provided that it is confined, should not preclude major intervention, as the first stage of this procedure is radical excision of any damaged tissue.

To highlight these principles, the authors have selected a series of 10 consecutive patients (see Table 7.1). The problem posed by the radiation damage—'frozen pelvis'—is demonstrated by Fig. 7.4. In this figure it can be clearly seen that, in addition to damage to the viscera with the development of fistulae, there is extensive fibrosis involving the pelvis, which can also result in constriction of the ureters. The principle of the first stage of this procedure, as mentioned above, is to excise completely all damaged tissue. A useful tip is to just uncap the ureter, as demonstrated in Fig. 7.4b, rather than completely skeletalizing it.

The surgical approach to these patients is, therefore, best considered as a two-stage procedure. The first stage is the radical excision of fibrotic and damaged tissue, the freeing of bowel adhesions and the resection of damaged pelvic viscera, including the rectum, bladder and vaginal remnants with the associated fistulous tracts. Adequate surgical access is mandatory and will usually necessitate an abdominoperineal approach. In

Age (years)	Diagnosis	Procedure
45	VVF*	AP† repair
70	VVF, rectal stenosis	AP repair and colo-anal repair
58	VVF, shrunken bladder	AP repair, caecocolocystoplasty
55	Vesicorectovaginal fistula	AP repair, pelvic exenteration
28	VVF, end colostomy	Colo-anal anastomosis, caecocystoplasty, colocystoplasty
49	VVF, short vagina	Ileocaecocystoplasty, colovaginoplasty
40	Vesicovaginorectal fistula, shrunken bladder, colostomy	Ileocaecocystoplasty, colo-anal anastomosis
71	Vesicovaginorectal fistula	AP repair
27	VVF, post-AP resection, short vagina, shrunken bladder	Caecocolovaginoplasty, ileocaecocystoplasty
41	Cutaneovesicovaginorectal fistula	Colonic conduit, pelvic extenteration

Table 7.1. Series of 10 consecutive patients presenting with sequelae of postirradiation pelvic injury
*VVF, vesicovaginal fistula.
†AP, abdominoperineal.

order to carry out this surgery efficiently it is necessary for the surgeon to be experienced in all aspects of pelvic surgery. Access is hampered by the implementation of any approach that views the pelvis as a series of vertical compartments, namely urological, gynaecological and colorectal. There is nothing worse, in these circumstances, than a 'committee' approach to the surgery (apart from other factors, there is often a problem with adequate surgical access). Secondly, having excised the damaged tissue, it is necessary to carry out a functional restoration of the pelvis (see Table 7.2).

The clinical problem posed by such patients is demonstrated in Figs 7.5 and 7.6, with operative views as seen in Fig 7.7. However, having excised all the damaged tissue, as demonstated in Fig. 7.4b, one achieves the so-called 'see through' pelvis (see Fig. 7.8). Subsequent reconstruction of each of the compartments is certainly very feasible. The individual aspects of the reconstructive procedures involved are considered in more detail below.

1. Restoration of bowel continuity
2. Reconstruction of the vagina
3. Augmentation of the bladder
4. Sphincter function
5. Filling of the dead space

Table 7.2. The principal aspects to be considered in functional restoration of the pelvis

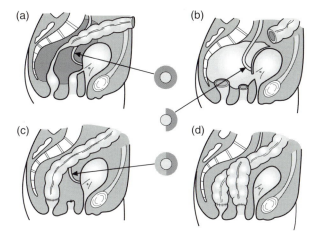

Figure 7.4. (a) Radiation-damaged pelvis with rectal stenosis, marked pelvic fibrosis, encasement of the ureter with fibrosis and a vesicovaginal fistula. (b) Excision of the damaged fibrotic tissue, including the abnormal rectum and vagina, with uncapping of the ureter. (c) Omental interposition and colo-anal anastomosis. Overclosure of the defect in the bladder. (d) Vaginal augmentation with caecocolovaginoplasty.

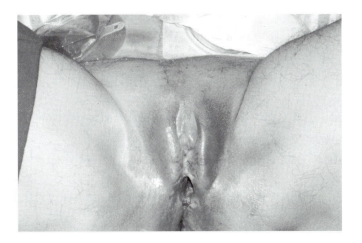

Figure 7.5. Patient with an irradiation-damaged pelvis who had previously undergone both a faecal and urinary diversion but is still left with a chronically discharging vulva.

Restoration of bowel continuity

Whenever possible, it is worth restoring bowel continuity, if necessary by a colo-anal anstomosis. This can easily be carried out because of the good access produced during the preliminary dissection. Surprisingly, in the authors' experience, the anal sphincter mechanism is rarely damaged by radiotherapy for gynaecological malignancy. These patients do heal slowly and hence it is worth carrying out a defunctioning procedure. The authors have found that a loop ileostomy is easy to perform, is well tolerated by the

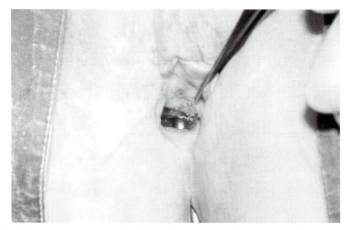

Figure 7.6. The same patient as in Fig. 7.5, demonstrating the presence of a rectovaginal fistula.

(a)

(b)

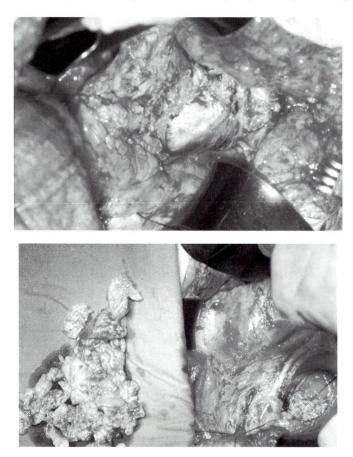

Figure 7.7. (a) Perioperative view of an irradiation-damaged pelvis, looking down into the pelvis from the cephalad position. The white tissue seen in the middle of the picture represents marked fibrosis within the pelvis. (b) Following excision of the fibrosis, a ureter with a ureteric catheter in situ can be seen. Part of the excised fibrotic tissue is in evidence on the right.

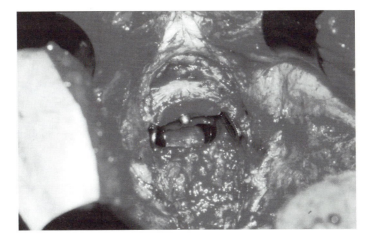

Figure 7.8. In this patient the bladder, vagina and rectum have been excised, producing the so-called 'see through' pelvis. Moving from the top of the figure to the bottom, a sound can be seen in the urethra, with a speculum behind this in the vaginal stump and a further one behind this in the anal canal.

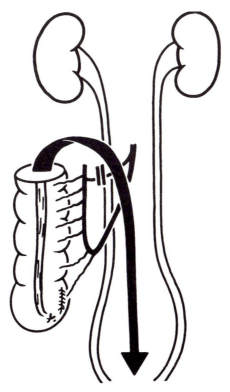

Figure 7.9. The use of the right colonic segment, including the caecum and ascending colon up to the hepatic flexure, produces a very capacious neovagina and, provided that an adequate length is taken, it easily reaches down to the vaginal stump to allow a tension-free anastomosis.

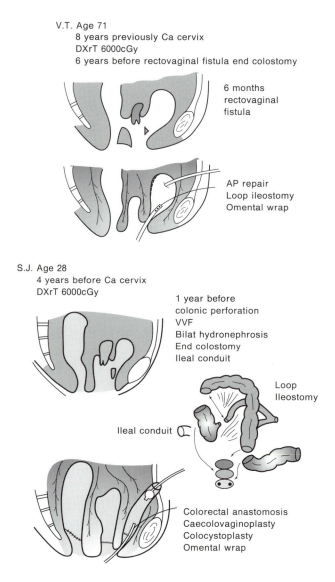

(a)

V.T. Age 71
8 years previously Ca cervix
DXrT 6000cGy
6 years before rectovaginal fistula end colostomy

6 months
rectovaginal
fistula

AP repair
Loop ileostomy
Omental wrap

(b)

S.J. Age 28
4 years before Ca cervix
DXrT 6000cGy

1 year before
colonic perforation
VVF
Bilat hydronephrosis
End colostomy
Ileal conduit

Loop
Ileostomy

Ileal conduit

Colorectal anastomosis
Caecolovaginoplasty
Colocystoplasty
Omental wrap

Figure 7.10. (a) A 71-year-old lady with a 6-month history of a rectovesicovaginal fistula, who underwent excision of damaged tissue, overclosure of the fistula and elimination of dead space by the interposition of omentum. (b) A 28-year-old lady with a vesicovaginal fistula and a past history of colonic perforation and with bilateral hydronephrosis, who had previously undergone an end colostomy and formation of an ileal conduit. A repair was carried out with a colo-anal anastomosis, caecocolovaginoplasty and a colocystoplasty brought out as a cutaneous conduit to allow 'bladder cycling', to test the integrity of the urethral sphincter mechanism. (c) (opposite) A 40-year-old lady with an obstructed left kidney, small-capacity bladder and a vesicovaginorectal fistula, who had previously undergone a Hartmann's procedure managed successfully with a colo-anal anastomosis and caecocystoplasty with a uretero-ileal anastomosis. (d) (opposite) A 41-year-old lady with a cutaneovesicovaginorectal fistula. The damaged tissue in the pelvis was excised, allowing formation of an end colostomy and a colonic urinary conduit in situ. There was marked improvement in the patient's quality of life.

(c)

M.C. Age 40
18 months before Ca cervix
Wertheim DXrT 5600cGy

Obstructed L. kidney
Small bladder
Double incontinent
Hartmanns procedure

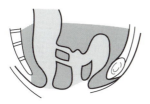

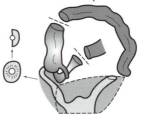

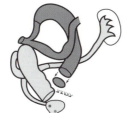

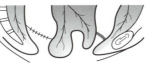

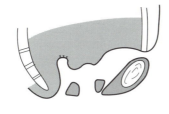

Colo-anal anastomosis
Caecocystoplasty
Uretero-ileal anastomosis
Omental wrap

1 year continent
Bladder capacity 450ml RU 50 ml

(d)

Age 41
3 years before cystadenocarcinoma Ovary
DXrT 5.500cGy

1 year before
rectosigmoid perforation

Small bowel - cutaneous
fistulae
2 laparotomies

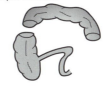

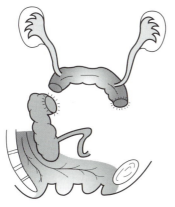

Colonic conduit
End colostomy
Omentoplasty

Fig. 10 (c) and (d), caption opposite.

patients and, in particular, usually uses bowel free of the irrradiated field, with resultant ease of closure and reduced morbidity.

Reconstruction of the vagina

In the relatively young age group it is obviously important to consider restoration of sexual function. The authors have found that the use of the right colonic segment is particularly advantageous in this context (Fig. 7.9). This produces a capacious vagina and is well tolerated by the patient, given adequate preoperative counselling (in particular, with regard to mucus production). Additionally, such a caecocolovaginoplasty has the benefit of contributing to abolition of dead space in the pelvis (Fig. 7.4d). The authors' experience with 13 patients treated with these vaginoplasties was reviewed recently.[44]

Augmentation of the bladder and consideration of sphincter function

Augmentation or substitution of the bladder is a standard part of the urologist's armamentarium; specific details relating to this are not, therefore, considered further here. In this context, particular consideration should be given to the fact that the urethral sphincter mechanism may well be impaired as a consequence of radiation injury. It is, therefore, worth while, in those patients where such a possibility is considered likely, to construct the subsequent neobladder in such a manner that a subsequent diversion (either continent or incontinent) can easily be carried out.

Filling dead space

Once all the tissue has been excised, it is clear from the above that a large raw area is produced within the pelvis and it is essential to the success of the overall procedure that this area is filled with vascularized tissue. As mentioned above, a neovaginal augmentation can be used to great advantage in this context. The authors have found, however, that, invariably, the omentum must be deployed. The principles of this are described in the first part of this chaper. Other authors have reported the use of musculocutaneous flaps.[39] Such techniques do, however, require specialist training and, unless there is extensive loss of the abdominal wall or peritoneal tissues, are not necessary, in the authors' experience. In addition, they have found that striated muscle, when introduced into the closed pelvis in the presence of devascularization, is more prone to infective complications than is omentm.

Discussion

It should be emphasized that such cases are extremely uncommon and that complex and invasive surgery is not appropriate for every case. Surgery in these patients is not without complication and will often require an extensive postoperative sojourn in hospital. Nevertheless, in selected cases a very satisfactory result can be achieved, with remarkable improvement in the patient's quality of life. The basic principles applied to the management of the patients are fundamental to surgery in general, namely (a) the excision of damaged devascularized tissue, (b) the interposition of vascularized tissue for reconstruction with the elimination of dead space, and (c) the temporary defunctioning of both the urinary and faecal streams. The cases illustrated in Fig. 7.10 illustrate representative case reports where a successful repair procedure was possible, yet highlighting that this is not possible in all cases (Fig. 7.10d).

In tackling this form of surgery, a comprehensive training in pelvic surgery is essential, as every case will be different and will require the implementation of different surgical techniques. Furthermore, it must be appreciated that the actual reconstruction procedure that is necessary will not be evident until the first part of the operation—namely, excision of the damaged tissue—has been completed.

References

1. Marshall V F. Vesicovaginal fistulas on one urological service. J Urol 1979; 121: 25–29
2. Collins C G, Pent D, Jones F B. Results of early repair of vesicovaginal fistula with preliminary cortisone treatment. Am J Obstet Gynecol 1960; 80: 1005
3. Lawson J. The management of genitourinary fistulae. Clin Obstet Gynecol 1987; 5: 209–236
4. O'Conor V J. Review of experience with vesicovaginal fistula repair. Trans Am Assoc Genitourin Surg 1979; 71: 120–122
5. Jonas U, Petri E. Genitourinary fistulae. In: Stanton S L (ed) Clinical gynaecological urology. St Louis: C V Mosby, 1984
6. Turner-Warwick R T. Repair of urinary vaginal fistulae. In: Innes-Williams D (ed) Urology. London: Butterworths, 1977; 206–218
7. Persky L, Herman G, Guerrier K. Non-delay in vesicovaginal fistula repair. Urology 1979; 13: 273–275
8. Badenoch D F, Tiptaft R C, Thakar D R et al. Early repair of accidental injury to the ureter or bladder following gynaecological surgery. Br J Urol 1987; 59: 516–518
9. Cruikshank S H. Early closure of posthysterectomy vesicovaginal fistulas. South Med J 1988; 81: 1525–1528
10. Roen P R. Combined vaginal and transvesical approach in successful repair of vesicovaginal fistula. Arch Surg 1960; 80: 628–633
11. Wayrauch H W, Rous S N. Transvesical-transvaginal approach for surgical repair of vesicovaginal fistulae. Surg Gynecol Obstet 1966; 123: 121–125
12. Douglas M. Operative treatment of urinary incontinence. Am J Obstet Gynecol 1936; 31: 268–279
13. Garlock J H. The cure of an intractable vesico-vaginal fistula by the use of a pedicled muscle flap. Surg Gynecol Obstet 1928; 47: 255–260
14. Ingleman-Sundberg. In: Meigs J V (ed) Surgical treatment of carcinoma of the cervix. London: Heinemann, 1954: 419
15. Hamlin R H J, Nicholson E C. Reconstruction of urethra totally destroyed in labour. Br Med J 1969; 2: 147–150
16. McCraw J B, Massey F M, Shanklin K D, Horton C E. Vaginal reconstruction with gracilis myocutaneous flaps. Plast Reconstr Surg 1976; 58: 176–183
17. Martius H. Die operative wiederherstellung der volkommen fehlenden harnrohre und der schliessmuskels derselben. Zentralbl Gynakol 1928; 52: 480–486

18. Spence H M, Duckett J W. Diverticulum of the female urethra: clinical aspects and presentation of a simple operative technique for cure. J Urol 1970; 104: 432–437
19. Turner-Warwick R T. The use of pedicle grafts in the repair of urinary tract fistulae. Br J Urol 1972; 44: 644–656
20. Zacharin R G. Grafting as a principle in the surgical management of vesico-vaginal and recto-vaginal fistulae. Aust N Z J Obstet Gynaecol 1980; 20: 10–17
21. O'Conor V J, Sokol J K, Bulkley G J, Nanninga J B. Suprapubic closure of vesicovaginal fistula. J Urol 1973; 109: 51–54
22. Turner-Warwick R T. Urinary fistula in the female. In: Harrison J H (eds) Campbell's Urology, 5th ed. Philadelphia: Saunders, 1979, ch 85
23. Walters W. Transperitoneal repair of a vesico-vaginal fistula. Proc Staff Meet Mayo Clin 1935; 375–377
24. Chapple C R, Turner-Warwick R T. Traumatic lower urinary tract fistulae—abdominoperineal repair with pedicled omental interposition. J Urol 1990; 143: 328A
25. Turner Warwick R T. The omental repair of complex urinary fistulae. In: Gingel C, Abrams P (eds) Controversies and innovations in urological surgery. London: Springer-Verlag, 1988: ch 26
26. Bardescu N. Ein neues verfahren fur die operation der tiefen blasen-uterus-scheidenfisteln. Zentralbl Gynakol 1900; 24: 170–175
27. Eisen M, Jurkovic K, Altwein J E et al. Management of vesicovaginal fistulas with peritoneal flap interposition. J Urol 1974; 112: 195–198
28. Robertson C N, Riefkohl R, Webster G N. Use of the rectus abdominis muscle in urological reconstructive procedures. J Urol 1986; 135: 963–965
29. McCraw J B, Arnold P G. Atlas of muscle and myocutaneous flaps. Norfolk, Va: Hampton Press, 1986
30. Coleman J W, Albanese C, Marion D et al. Experimental use of free grafts of bladder mucosa in canine bladders—successful closure of recurrent vesicovaginal fistula utilising bladder mucosa. Urology 1985; 25: 515–517
31. Kiricuta I, Goldstein A M B. Epiplooplastia vezicula, metoda de tratament curativ al fistulelor vezico-vaginale. Obstet Ginecol Bucereste 1956; 2: 163–175
32. Turner-Warwick R T, Wynne E J C, Handley-Ashken M. The use of the omental pedicle graft in the repair and reconstruction of the urinary tract. Br J Surg 1967; 54: 849–853
33. Goldstein M B, Dearden L C. Histology of omentoplasty of the urinary bladder in the rabbit. Invest Urol 1966; 3: 460–469
34. Helmbrecht L J, Goldstein A M B, Morrow J W. The use of pedicled omentum in the repair of large vesicovaginal fistulas. Invest Urol 1975; 13: 104–107
35. Kiricuta L, Goldstein A M B. The repair of extensive vesicovaginal fistulas with pedicled omentum. J Urol 1972; 108: 724–727
36. Chapple C R, Turner-Warwick R T. Surgical salvage of radiation induced fibrosis—the 'frozen pelvis'. J Urol 1990; 143: 349A
37. Turner-Warwick R T, Kirby R S. Principles of sphincteroplasty. In: Webster G D, Goldwasser B, King L, Kirby R (eds) Reconstructive urology. Boston: Blackwell, 1992: 657–686
38. Eddington H D, Sugarbaker P H, McDonald H G. Management of the surgically traumatised irradiated and infected pelvis. Surgery 1988; 103: 692–697
39. Mathes S J, Hurwitz D J. Repair of chronic radiation wounds to the pelvis. World J Surg 1986; 10: 269–280
40. Borkowski A, Nowacki M. Simultaneous repair of post-irradiation vesico-vaginal and recto-vaginal fistulas. J Urol 192; 128: 926–928
41. van Nagell J R, Parker J, Maruyama Y et al. Bladder or rectal injury following radiation therapy for cervical cancer. Am J Obstet Gynecol 1974; 119: 727–732
42. Jakowatz J G, Porudominsky D, Riihimaki D U et al. Complications of pelvic exenteration. Arch Surg 1985; 120: 1261–1265
43. Ckrause S, Hald T, Steven K. Surgery for urological complications following radiotherapy for gynaecologic cancer. Scand J Urol Nephrol 1987; 21: 115–118
44. Turner-Warwick R T, Kirby R S. The construction and reconstruction of the vagina with the colo-caecum. Surg Gynecol Obstet 1990; 170: 132–136

Sexual function after pelvic radiotherapy

8

V. Beckendorf and le Groupe Urologie de la
CMIC–FNCLCC   A. Schwander-Lesur
M.-P. Mayeur   I. Pouchard

Introduction

After pelvic radiotherapy it has been noted that the mechanisms, the frequency and the impact of modification of sexual function differ widely between male and female patients. The types of tumours treated by radiotherapy with a curative intent are mainly urological in men and occur after 60 years of age: these are cancers of the prostate and, less often, urinary bladder cancer. The main problem is to allow normal erectile and ejaculatory function. In women, gynaecological tumours predominate and can occur before 40 years of age, when reproductive and hormonal function are severely impaired. The difficulties involve hormonal status, libido and dyspareunia.

This chapter reports the results of a recent prospective multicentre study of sexual function in 67 men treated for prostatic carcinoma. Discussion of the situation in female patients is based on an analysis of two retrospective studies in women treated either with a combination of radiotherapy and surgery, or with radiotherapy alone, for cancer of the cervix.

Evolution of sexual function after prostate cancer radiotherapy

A prospective study was performed in five French Departments of Radiation Oncology to assess the evolution of sexual function after curative radiotherapy of prostatic carcinoma. For the French population, there is only one recent retrospective study based on a mailed questionnaire.[1] Other studies have reported 50–80% preservation of potency after external beam irradiation; with nerve-sparing radical retropubic prostatectomy, potency can be expected to range from 50 to 75%.[2–5] Over the past few years, the age of the population treated by radiotherapy has been increasing, as has the practice of prostatectomy.

The study started in January 1992 in five centres. Different urological trends and radiotherapy techniques were encountered, depending on the centre, and reflecting usual practices.

The treatment of the tumour and its evolution were described and recorded for each patient as well as his medical history. Any drug-taking,[6] social activity, existence of a partner and psychological impact of cancer were also noted. The main part of the study was a further questionnaire reviewing libido, nightly or morning erections, frequency of sexual activity, quality of erection to start, continue and achieve coition, ejaculation, pleasure or satisfaction. As psychogenic factors can be responsible for sexual disorders, it was decided not to investigate men who did not complain of any problem. A series of examinations was designed for patients wishing to have a problem investigated of which they were already aware.[7]

Sixty-seven patients were followed up more than 10 months after the end of radiotherapy, when subacute secondary effects had subsided and questionnaires were available. Another questionnaire was planned at the end of the second year after treatment when fibrosis and sequelae had become established. The patients' ages ranged from 54 to 84 years with an average of 68 years; 63 were married and 50 had an active partner. In 42 cases, there was another previous pathological condition for which the medical treatment was able to induce sexual dysfunction; however, performance status and life expectancy ranged from good to excellent.

Of the 67 patients, 13 had stage A disease, 44 stage B and 10 stage C. All patients received definitive external beam irradiation with 25 MV X-rays at dose levels ranging from 58 to 70 Gy with a mean dose of 68 Gy. Five received a short initial hormone treatment. At the time of follow-up, there was no clinical cancer relapse, but two patients showed an increase in prostate-specific antigen (PSA). Four patients had received prolonged hormonal treatment, without explanation in two cases. One patient died of another cause.

Before radiotherapy, 40 had sexual activity with good to satisfactory intercourse. The same proportion of men with sexual activity was observed in the various age groups, but the frequency of sexual intercourse decreased with age. Professional activity and active retirement, often linked to younger age and good performance status, were associated with continued sexual activity. Tumour stage, PSA level, transurethral resection or lymphadenectomy, other pathology and initial hormonal status had no effect on sexual activity before treatment.

Comparison of the various aspects of sexual function before and after prostatic irradiation showed that libido was the best preserved (90%). At the interview it was claimed that the other aspects were preserved to a degree of 64–75%. Since potency involves more than a nightly erection, effective conservation of sexual function was defined as when the patient had a full erection, or at least partial erection adequate for coitus with satisfaction, and sexual intercourse a few times before the interview if there was an existing partner. In this respect, function was retained in 72% of cases, but only 21 of 40 patients reported no change (Table 8.1).

Function	No. of patients with function		Percentage preservation of function
	Before RTH*	After RTH	
Libido	47	43	90
Nightly or morning erection	50	32	64
Full erection	42	27	67
Sexual intercourse before therapy	40	29	72
Monthly frequency of intercourse	1–12 (mean 5.5)	1–10 (mean 3.7)	
Satisfaction	32	24	75

Table 8.1. *Sexual function before and after radiotherapy in 67 male patients*
*RTH, radiotherapy.

Factors that gave a good prognosis for preservation of function included age (especially for the frequency of intercourse) and monthly frequency of intercourse before treatment, with a marked difference between patients claiming a frequency of more than three and those claiming less. None of the patients with only partial erection achieved preservation of function (Table 8.2). In this study, some factors had no predictive value: these included tumour stage, radiation dose, associated pathologies such as vascular or urological disease, and drugs inducing sexual dysfunction. Several possible causes of impairment of sexual function were probably associated.

Factor	No. of patients	Preservation of function*	Frequency of intercourse (no./month)	
			Before RTH†	After RTH
Age at treatment:				
≤68	36	12/17 (71)	4.8	4.4
≥69	31	17/23 (74)	4.8	1.8
Social activity:				
Professional activity	7	5/6 (83)		
Active retirement	52	23/31 (74)		
Minimal activity	8	1/3 (33)		
Monthly frequency of intercourse before treatment:				
>3	27	19/27 (70)	5.8	4.3
1–3	13	5/13 (38)	2.1	1.5
Erection quality before treatment:				
Partial erection	8	0/8 (0)		

Table 8.2. *Preservation of sexual function in male patients receiving radiotherapy: factors of prognostic value*

*No. of patients, with percentages in parentheses.
†RTH, radiotherapy.

It was concluded that the rate of preservation of potency and sexual activity after 1 year was the same as in other studies, depending on definitions [1, 8–12] (Table 8.3). Only a few patients demanded investigation or treatment for dysfunction, although many had a real problem. The choice of a partner may therefore be important; perhaps, in some cases, the partner was not sufficiently stimulating.

Author and year	No. of patients	Mean age (years)	No. of patients sexually active before RTH*	Percentage of patients sexually active after RTH†
Bagshaw et al. (1988)[8]	914	63	434	86 (15 months) 50 (7 years)
Banker (1988)[9]	85	64–68	85	54 (1 year)
Van Heeringen et al. (1988)[10]	18	71	12	25
Zinreich et al. (1990)[11]	27	68	10	30 (1 year)
Berger et al. (1993)[1]	56	64	44	59 (1 year)

Table 8.3. Studies of sexual function following radiotherapy of the prostate
*RTH, radiotherapy.
†Duration of follow-up in parentheses.

Evolution of sexual function after treatment of cervical cancer

Two retrospective studies were carried out in Nancy[13] and Lyon[14] on 100 women treated for cervical cancer, either by combined radiotherapy and surgery, or by radiotherapy alone, between 1981 and 1985. All patients received 60 Gy by endobrachytherapy; 35 had external beam irradiation to the pelvis, delivering between 20 and 50 Gy; 80 had undergone hysterectomy. The mean age was 46 years. Tumour stage was T_{is} in five cases, T_{1a} in 22, T_{1b} in 49 and T_2 in 24. The studies were based on written questionnaires, interviews and clinical examinations, with an average delay of 3 years after treatment. All women were free of disease at the time of the study.

Before treatment, 17 women had no partner and 25 were menopausal. In 30%, the first signs of cancer, investigations and diagnosis induced modifications of sexual activity.

The most important and constant consequence of irradiation for young women was the premature onset of the menopause, 12–15 Gy being sufficient to induce menopause, depending on the age of the patient. In this series, only 30 patients received hormone replacement therapy and the usual troubles of menopause were compounded by the direct effects of radiation. The gynaecological tumour, the loss of fertility and the menopause were described as reducing their femininity by 43% of patients.

After treatment, eight women no longer had any sexual activity. The length and breadth of the vaginal cavity had shrunk in 22% and severe vaginal stenosis occurred in 7%. Vaginal dryness was reported in 70 cases and dyspareunia occurred in 57%. Some women had postcoital bleeding; although this was not severe, it always gave rise to anxiety. Sexual activity was resumed 1–3 months after treatment in half the cases.

According to the questionnaires, there was a decrease of libido in 40% of patients, of sexual frequency in 42% and of sexual satisfaction in 47%.

Half the women (50%) admitted to fearing a recurrence of the tumour or pain, blaming their sexuality for their condition. Besides sexual dysfunction, problems occurred with the partner, who in some cases found another partner or separated. More than half the women thought that better information would have helped them.[15]

This study focused on low-stage cervical cancer; any anatomical modification of the vagina is likely to be more severe in stage III cancer (Table 8.4). The larger the tumours, the more severe the pelvic sequelae. Treatment of endometrial cancer is associated with fewer changes.[16] As is the case for other aspects, improvement of radiation dosimetry can reduce the rate of complications after treatment.

Author and year	Vaginal changes	Reduced libido	Reduced satisfaction	Reduced frequency
Vincent et al. (1975)[17]			24	29
Seibel et al. (1980)[18]	37			76
Bruner et al. (1993)[16]	18		37	22
Cull et al. (1993)[15]		49	47	47

Table 8.4. Studies of sexual function following radiotherapy of gynaecological tumours*
*Values are percentages.

Discussion and conclusions

The sequelae of radiotherapy on sexual function are difficult to evaluate. In men, problems of sterility are minor, no study of the semen quality has been undertaken after prostatic or vesical irradiation. The testes receive only low doses and spermatogenesis may be delayed but not completely inhibited. The hormonal status is unaltered. The major problem is impotence and the ability to achieve erection, penetration and completion of intercourse. Difficulties depend on the urological management.

In women, fertility and hormonal status are the main problems and hormonal treatment can partly compensate for this. In recent studies, 10% of patients have claimed improved sexuality after treatment. Anatomical modifications more often affect satisfaction than capacity for sexual activity, as only less than 10% vaginal stenosis is observed and necrosis no longer occurs. Vaginal dilators, lubricating creams and recommendation of an early return to intercourse can help patients.[19]

In all cases, information about the secondary effects of treatment and their management must be given. Psychogenic factors are often associated with physical changes and, in some cases, require particular management.[10,11,12,15]

Acknowledgements

We thank Professor J. Leclère, Professor P. Mangin and Dr M. J. Grillot from the Departments of Endocrinology, Urology, and Rehabilitation, Centre Hospitalier Universitaire de Brabois, Vandoeuvre-les-Nancy, France, for their suggestions regarding the preparation of the prostate questionnaire.

References

1. Berger C, Rocher F P, Zhu Y et al. Activité sexuelle après irradiation pelvienne pour cancer de la prostate. J Urol (Paris) 1993; 99: 219–227
2. Catalona W J, Basler J W. Return of erections and urinary continence following nerve sparing radical retropubic prostatectomy. J Urol 1993; 150: 905–907
3. Drago J R, Badalament R A, York J P et al. Radical prostatectomy: OSU and affiliated hospitals' experience 1985–1989. Urology 1992; 39: 44–47
4. Leandri P, Rossignol G, Gautier J R, Ramon J. Radical retropubic prostatectomy: morbidity and quality of life. Experience with 620 consecutive cases. J Urol 1992; 147: 883–887
5. Quinlan D M, Epstein J I, Carter B S, Walsh P C. Sexual function following radical prostatectomy: influence of preservation of neurovascular bundles. J Urol 1991; 145: 998–1002
6. Médicaments provocant des troubles sexuels (ML USA 744), Med Lett Drugs Ther 1987; 9(17): 73–76
7. Krane R J, Goldstein I, Saenz de Tejada I. Impotence. N Engl J Med 1989; 321: 1648–1659
8. Bagshaw M A, Cox R S, Ray G R. Status of radiation treatment of prostate cancer at Stanford University. NCI Monogr 1988; 7: 47–60
9. Banker F L. The preservation of potency after external beam irradiation for prostate cancer. Int J Radiat Oncol Biol Phys 1988; 15: 219–220
10. Van Heeringen C, De Schryver A, Verbeek E. Sexual function disorders after local radiotherapy for carcinoma of the prostate. Radiother Oncol 1988; 13: 47–52
11. Zinreich E S, Derogatis L R, Herpst J et al. Pretreatment evaluation of sexual function in patients with adenocarcinoma of the prostate. Int J Radiat Oncol Biol Phys 1990; 19: 1001–1004

12. Zinreich E S, Derogatis L R, Herpst J et al. Pre- and post-treatment evaluation of sexual function in patients with adenocarcinoma of the prostate. Int J Radiat Oncol Biol Phys 1990; 19: 729–732

13. Mayeur M P. Le gynécologue face aux conséquences des traitements des cancers du col de l'utérus. Analyse de 131 cas traités au Centre Alexis Vautrin. [thèse] Nancy (F): Université de Nancy I, 1988

14. Brune-Pouchard I. Evaluation de l'activité sexuelle après traitement du cancer du col utérin. [mémoire] Lyon (F): Université Claude-Bernard Lyon I, 1986

15. Cull A, Cowie V J, Farquharson D I et al. Early stage cervical cancer: psychosocial and sexual outcomes of treatment. Br J Cancer 1993; 68: 1216–1220

16. Bruner D W, Lanciano R, Keegan M et al. Vaginal stenosis and sexual function following intracavitary radiation for the treatment of cervical and endometrial carcinoma. Int J Radiat Oncol Biol Phys 1993; 27: 825–830

17. Vincent C E, Vincent B, Greiss F C, Linton E B. Some marital–sexual concomitants of carcinoma of the cervix. South Med J 1975; 68: 552–558

18. Seibel M M, Freemann M G, Graves W L. Carcinoma of the cervix and sexual function. Obstet Gynecol 1980; 55: 484–487

19. Schwander-Lesur A, Mayeur M P, Guillemin F. Les séquelles urologiques, gynécologiques et endocriniennes des traitements du cancer du col de l'utérus chez 131 femmes âgées de moins de 50 ans Contracept Fertil Sexual 1990; 18: 45–49

Erectile dysfunction after genitourinary pelvic surgery

9

S. B. Radomski   M. S. Liquornik

Introduction

In the general population, approximately 20% of men over the age of 50 are impotent. Common causes responsible for this are vascular disease, diabetes and medication. Patients undergoing any pelvic surgery are at risk of developing impotence postoperatively. The presence of vascular disease, diabetes and medication may enhance the risk significantly. This review examines erectile dysfunction as a complication of genitourinary pelvic surgery and its treatment in this group of patients.

Physiology of erection

Penile erection is a complex neurovascular phenomenon involving the specific haemodynamic events of increased arterial flow and decreased venous drainage, as well as the interaction of nerves, neurotransmitters, striated and smooth muscle, and the tunica albuginea. The key to the erectile process is the cavernous smooth muscles and the smooth muscle of the arterial wall. In erection, there is relaxation of these smooth muscles allowing for (a) sinusoidal relaxation, (b) arterial dilatation and, therefore, increased blood flow and (c) venous compression and the resulting decrease in venous outflow.

Penile blood supply

The penile blood supply is bilateral and is derived from the pudendal artery, which is a branch of the internal iliac artery. The pudendal artery forms three end-arteries to supply the penis—the dorsal penile artery, the cavernous artery and the bulbourethral artery. Venous drainage of the penis is extensive and controversial. The sinusoids, which are a sponge-like blood-filled trabeculated network filling the corporal bodies, drain into the emissary veins, which in turn drain into the deep dorsal and cavernous veins; these veins then drain into the pudendal veins. Other veins involved in the drainage of the proximal corpus spongiosum include the bulbar and urethral veins. There is much crossover between veins draining the penis, making this a very complex system.

Penile innervation

Both the autonomic and somatic nervous systems are involved in the erectile process.

The autonomic nervous system involves both parasympathetic and sympathetic nerves, which merge to form the cavernosal nerve that innervates the penis. The parasympathetic system, which is thought to be of primary importance in erection, has neurons in the interomediolateral cell columns of S2–4 that contribute fibres to the pelvic nerve. The pelvic nerve travels within the endopelvic fascia and joins the pelvic plexus, found alongside the rectum, from which the cavernosal nerve arises, as does the innervation to other pelvic organs. The contribution of the sympathetic nervous system to erection is less fully elucidated. Neurons from the T11–L2 spinal cord levels contribute fibres to the superior hypogastric plexus, which then gives rise to the right and left hypogastric nerves. These hypogastric nerves then feed into the pelvic plexus from which the cavernosal nerve arises.

The somatic nervous system is responsible for the motor innervation of the bulbocavernosus and ischiocavernosus muscles via Onuf's nucleus in the S2–4 spinal cord, which gives fibres to the pudendal nerve which, in turn, innervates these muscles. The somatosensory pathway for the penis involves the dorsal nerve of the penis, the fibres of which enter the pudendal nerve, which then enters the spinal cord at the S2–4 level to continue via the spinothalamic tract to the cerebrum.

The neurotransmitters, and their absolute roles in the erectile state, have not been fully elucidated. Acetylcholine is involved in smooth muscle relaxation and is important but not exclusively responsible for erection. Many studies have suggested a non-adrenergic non-cholinergic involvement. Other transmitters that are involved in the erectile process include nitric oxide, prostaglandins and vasoactive intestinal polypeptide, to name but a few. Nitric oxide, which acts via a cGMP mechanism to induce smooth muscle relaxation, is now considered the most likely candidate for the principal neurotransmitter in erection.[1]

Pelvic surgery

Erectile dysfunction can result from any alteration in any one of the components outlined above that are involved in the complex process of erection. This chapter focuses on the effects of pelvic surgery on the erectile process. The aetiology of erectile dysfunction can be divided, be means of the 'functional classification of erectile dysfunction', into neurogenic, vasculogenic, psychogenic and hormonal categories. Pelvic surgery, if responsible for erectile dysfunction, leads to erectile dysfunction primarily by affecting the nerves or blood vessels that are involved in the erectile process. Psychogenic factors can certainly be involved as a result of the psychological stresses of undergoing major operations, often for malignant or life-threatening ailments, but this topic is not extensively discussed in this chapter.

There are scores of different pelvic surgical procedures that are associated with erectile dysfunction as a side effect. These include genitourinary operations such as prostatectomy, cystectomy and retroperitoneal lymph node dissection. General surgical operations that can lead to erectile dysfunction include abdominal perineal resections, low anterior resections, pelvic exenterations and others. Vascular operations that can result in erectile dysfunction include aortobifemoral bypasses, abdominal aortic aneurysmal resections and others.

Benign prostate disease surgery

The mechanism of erectile dysfunction after prostatectomy for benign disease is unclear. Age and preoperative sexual function appear to be important underlying factors that determine postprostatectomy impotence. It appears that many men who develop impotence after prostatectomy have underlying erectile dysfunction preoperatively.[2,3] Patients over the age of 60 have an increased risk of impotence after prostatectomy.[4,5] Suprapubic or retropubic prostatectomy for benign disease has been reported to result in a 14–25% rate of impotence, compared with 4% for transurethral resection.[6,7] However, in a recent study comparing transurethral prostatectomy with watchful waiting, 19% of the men in the surgery group and 21% in the watchful-waiting group reported that their sexual per-formance was worse.[8] Other authors feel that there is no significant differ-ence between the suprapubic/retropubic approach and the transurethral approach.[3] The suprapubic/retropubic prostatectomy can theoretically result in injury to the neurovascular structures important for erection. Injury to the neurovascular bundles posterolaterally on the prostatic capsule can occur by the actual incision or by tearing of this capsular incision. Furthermore, aggressive cauterization and suturing of bleeders may result in injury to the neurovascular bundles.

The many newer alternatives to standard prostate surgery, which include the use of a laser, electrocautery vaporization and thermotherapy, also have an incidence of erectile dysfunction. As no long-term data are yet available, the exact numbers are not known; however, the rates of impotence do not seem to be higher than that for the standard transurethral resection of the prostate and, in fact, are reported to be lower.[9]

Psychogenic factors may also play a significant role in causing postprostatectomy impotence.[10] Many believe that a psychogenic aetiology is more likely than an organic aetiology for erectile dysfunction after simple prostatectomy. Patients who are well informed and who have a good general mental outlook on life preoperatively seem to do better with regard to potency status postoperatively.[10]

Radical prostatectomy

It is well documented throughout the urological literature that impotence is a common sequela of radical prostatectomy. Age of the patient and preoperative sexual function are also key factors in postoperative potency status, as for simple prostatectomy. It is believed that the increased rate of impotence after radical prostatectomy for prostate cancer is the result of injury to the pelvic nerves which, as described above, travel as a neurovascular bundle within the endopelvic fascia closely adherent to both the rectum and the prostate gland at the posterolateral aspect. Walsh and Donker (1982) initially reported that impotence during radical prosta-tectomy resulted from injury to the autonomic nerves during dissection of the apex of the prostate or during dissection of the lateral pelvic fascia and pedicle.[11] Walsh and Mostwin (1984) described a nerve-sparing technique whereby these nerves are preserved during the operation and an 80% or greater potency rate is obtained.[12]

However, some controversy exists as to the success of such a nerve-sparing approach on potency. The success, as mentioned, is also confound-ed by preoperative erectile dysfunction, age and psychological factors. If both neurovascular bundles are preserved, potency rates range from 42 to 86% at 1 year postoperatively.[12–14] If only one neurovascular bundle is preserved, potency rates range from 30 to 56%.[13] These potency rates appear to be higher in men under the age of 60.[15] Quinlan et al. (1991) reported that the potency rates in men over the age of 70, with both neuro-vascular bundles spared, was only 22%.[13]

Another potential cause of erectile dysfunction after radical prostatect-omy includes injury or ligation of the obturator or vesical arteries or their branches. This factor may be even more significant in patients with pre-operative vascular disease. The number of patients after radical prostat-ectomy who suffer from impotence as the result of this vascular aetiology is not well documented.

Radical cystoprostatectomy and urethrectomy

Radical cystoprostatectomy without urethrectomy is essentially similar to a radical prostatectomy with regard to the technique of sparing the neurovascular bundles for potency. Results in terms of potency are again similar. When a urethrectomy is added to the procedure, further care must be taken to preserve the cavernous nerves. Brendler et al. (1990) described the technique of preserving these nerves during urethrectomy.[16] They felt that injury to the cavernous nerves during urethrectomy occurred during mobilization of the membranous portion of the urethra, as the nerves course posterolaterally.[16]

Vascular surgery

DePalma et al. (1978) reported a 21–88% impotence rate after aorto-iliac revascularization in men who were potent preoperatively.[17] The pro-posed aetiology for this erectile dysfunction includes injury to the autonomic nerves, described above, and/or disturbance or interruption of adequate pelvic blood flow.[18] DePalma (1982) described a nerve-sparing technique, to be utilized during infrarenal aortic surgery, that reduces the incidence of postoperative impotence.[19] Kempczinski and Birinyi (1985) emphasize that, in order to preserve erectile function, surgery for aorto-iliac disease must minimize disturbance of genital autonomic nerves and maintain adequate pelvic blood flow.[20] These authors emphasize that preservation of adequate perfusion into a minimum of one hypogastric artery is of vital importance if iatrogenic erectile dysfunction is to be minimized.

It should be noted that, as up to 80% of patients who present with aorto-iliac occlusive disease have erectile dysfunction, the operative procedure that follows the above principles and allows for hypogastric artery perfusion can relieve erectile dysfunction in up to 30% of patients.[18,21]

Surgery for large bowel disease

Erectile dysfunction after sigmoid–rectal–anal surgery is not uncommon and is also dependent on the age of the patient and the extent of the surgical dissection.[22,23] The incidence of impotence after an abdominal perineal resection is reported to be approximately 15%.[23] Other operations implicated in postoperative erectile dysfunction include low anterior resections and proctocolectomies.

Retroperitoneal lymph node dissection for testicular cancer

Retroperitoneal lymph node dissection for testicular cancer can result in either ejaculatory failure or retrograde ejaculation. This is the result of possible injury to the sympathetic fibres coming from the thoracolumbar outflow (T11–L3), which converge anterior to the aorta. They then pass bilaterally along the aortic bifurcation anterior to the common iliac arteries reaching the hypogastric plexus. These sympathetic nerves innervate the vas deferens, seminal vesicles, prostate and bladder neck. Recently, nerve-sparing techniques and a modification in the extent of the dissection have been used to preserve the sympathetic fibres during lymph node dissection.[24–26] This has resulted in preservation of ejaculation in more than 80% of these patients.[25–27]

Treatments

Medication

Yohimbine as a treatment for impotence is controversial. It may be helpful in some instances where libido is low or psychogenic causes are responsible for the erectile failure.[28–30] Positive response rates have been in the range of 42–62% but in some controlled studies results were no better than a placebo, statistically.[30,31] Yohimbine acts by an alpha-2 antagonist effect but this effect has not been proved to be responsible for its efficacy in the treatment of impotence. Its use in patients with a neurogenic or vasculogenic cause of their impotence, as is usually the case after pelvic surgery, is limited.

Psychological counselling

Psychological factors may, in the postoperative period, be a significant aetiological cause of impotence. Anxiety and fears related to the diagnosed disease, the operation and recovery, as well as altered body image, can all be contributory factors. If the diagnosis of psychogenic impotence is based on the history and physical examination and supported by tests, such as nocturnal penile tumescence testing, psychological counselling with an experienced sexual therapist using a variety of techniques, including behavioural therapy, is very effective.[32] It should be noted that, even if an organic aetiology is diagnosed, there are often psychological sequelae that may merit the help of a sex counsellor. The combination of psychological therapy with another form of treatment is often advantageous and quite effective.

Vacuum erectile device

Almost all patients who are impotent after pelvic surgery, regardless of aetiology, are candidates for a vacuum erectile device. Success and satis-faction rates are high.[33] The devices, however, require careful instruction as to their use, as well as good manual dexterity.

The erection obtained is secondary to penile engorgement resulting in a rigid penis distal to the constriction band. This fact, coupled with the lack of spontaneity, may be a cause for dislike and discontinuation of use among patients.

Self-intracorporeal injection therapy

Intracorporeal injection of pharmacological agents, which act primarily through a smooth muscle relaxant effect, is effective in most types of impotence.[34] The agents most commonly used are papaverine or prosta-glandin E1. Often, these agents in combination with phentolamine are used as a so-called 'triple P' mixture. Patients with vasculogenic impotence may not respond as well as other patients and may require larger doses; conversely, patients with neurogenic impotence often have a strong response to lower doses of these pharmacological agents. This is important to remember in patients who have erectile dysfunction after pelvic surgery as the aetiology of their problem is usually neurological, as described above. The minimum dose suitable for an erection is utilized, thus reducing the incidence of priapism, a prolonged erection, which is one of the potentially more devastating side effects of this form of therapy. Success rates and satisfaction rates with this form of therapy are high;[35] however, with time, high drop-out rates are reported.[36]

Penile prosthesis

Penile prostheses are a common form of treatment for erectile dysfunction in our society, especially in the patient after pelvic surgery. With the advent of self-injection therapy, placement of a penile prosthesis has usually been used as a second-line therapy. This is especially important, as the other therapeutic techniques described are reversible whereas prosthesis placement should be considered irreversible. Although success rates and satisfaction rates are high, reoperation rates up to 50% with older devices are described. With the more modern devices, reoperation rates of 5–10% at 5 years can be expected.[37]

Modern penile prostheses are of primarily two types—semi-rigid and inflatable. The type of prosthesis used is based primarily on patient and surgeon preference.

Conclusions

All patients undergoing genitourinary pelvic surgery are at risk of sexual dysfunction as a complication. This risk is enhanced by age and medical status. Increased knowledge of anatomy and improved surgical technique have reduced the incidence of this complication. Furthermore, effective and acceptable treatments are available in most instances.

References

1. Burnett A L, Lowenstein C J, Bredt D S et al. Nitric oxide: a physiological mediator of penile erection. Science 1992; 257: 401
2. Bolt J W, Evans C, Marshal V R. Sexual dysfunction after prostatectomy. Br J Urol 1986; 58: 319
3. Hargreave T B, Stephenson T P. Potency and prostatectomy. Br J Urol 1977; 49: 683
4. Finkle A L, Moyers T G. Sexual potency in aging males: status of private patients before and after prostatectomy. J Urol 1960; 84: 1952
5. Gold F M, Hotchkiss R S. Sexual potency following simple prostatectomy. N Y State J Med 1969; 69: 2987
6. Hauri D. Life after prostatectomy. Urol Int 1982; 37: 271
7. Finkle A L, Prian D V. Sexual potency in elderly men before and after prostatectomy. JAMA 1966; 196: 139
8. Wasson J H, Reda D J, Bruskewitz R C et al. A comparison of transurethral surgery with watchful-waiting for moderate symptoms of benign prostatic hyperplasia. N Engl J Med 1995; 332: 75
9. Kabalin J N, Gill H S, Bite G. Laser prostatectomy performed with a right angle firing neodymium:YAG laser fiber at 60 watts power setting. J Urol 1995; 153: 1502
10. Ozhar J, Meiraz D, Moaz B. Factors influencing sexual activity after prostatectomy: a prospective study. J Urol 1976; 116: 332
11. Walsh P C, Donker P J. Impotence following radical prostatectomy: insight into aetiology and prevention. J Urol 1982; 128: 492
12. Walsh P C, Mostwin J L. Radical prostatectomy and cystoprostatectomy with preservation of potency: results utilizing a new nerve sparing technique. Br J Urol 1984; 56: 694

13. Quinlan D M, Epstein J I, Carter B S et al. Sexual function following radical prostatectomy, influence of preservation of neurovascular bundles. J Urol 1991; 145: 998
14. Leach G E. Potency evaluated after radical retropubic prostatectomy. AUA 92 Clin Perspect 1992; 5: 1
15. Keetch D W, Andriole G L, Catalona W J. Complications of radical retropubic prostatectomy. AUA Update Ser 1994; 13: Lesson 6
16. Brendler C B, Schlegel P N, Walsh P C. Urethrectomy with preservation of potency. J Urol 1990; 144: 270
17. DePalma R G, Levine S B, Feldman S. Preservation of erectile function after aortoiliac reconstruction. Arch Surg 1978; 113: 958
18. Flanigan D P, Schuler J J, Kifer T et al. Elimination of iatrogenic impotence and improvement of sexual function after aortoiliac revascularization. Arch Surg 1982; 117: 544
19. DePalma R G. Impotence in vascular disease: relationship to vascular surgery. Br J Surg 1982; 69: 514
20. Kempczinski R F, Birinyi L K. Impotence following aortic surgery. In: Bernard V M, Towne J B (eds) Complications in vascular surgery. Orlando: Grune and Stratton, 1985; 311
21. May A G, DeWeese J A, Rob C J. Changes in sexual function following operation on the abdominal aorta. Surgery 1969; 65: 41
22. Weinstein M, Roberts M. Sexual potency following surgery for rectal carcinoma: a follow-up of 44 patients. Ann Surg 1977; 185: 295
23. Yeager E S, Van Heerden J A. Sexual dysfunction following proctocolectomy and abdominoperineal resection. Ann Surg 1980; 191: 169
24. Fossa S, Kleep O, Ous J et al. Unilateral retroperitoneal lymph node dissection in patients with nonseminomatous testicular tumour in clinical stage I. Eur Urol 1984; 10: 17
25. Donohue J, Foster R, Rowland R et al. Nerve-sparing retroperitoneal lymphadenectomy with preservation of ejaculation. J Urol 1990; 144: 287
26. Jewett M A S, Kong Y, Goldberg S et al. Retroperitoneal lymphadenectomy for testis tumour with nerve-sparing for ejaculation. J Urol 1988; 139: 1220
27. Colleselli K, Poisel S, Schachtner W, Bartsh G. Nerve-preserving bilateral retroperitoneal lymphadenectomy: anatomical study and operative approach. J Urol 1990; 144: 293
28. Riley A J, Goodman R E, Kellett J M, Orr R. Double-blind trial of yohimbine hydrochloride in the treatment of erection inadequacy. J Sex Marital Ther 1989; 4: 17
29. Sussett J G, Tessier C D, Wincze J et al. Effect of yohimbine hydrochloride on erectile impotence: a double-blind study. J Urol 1989; 141: 1360
30. Reid K, Morales A, Harris C et al. Double-blind trial of yohimbine in treatment of psychogenic impotence. Lancet 1987; 2: 421
31. Morales A, Surridge D H, Marshall P G, Fenmore J. Non-hormonal pharmacological treatment of organic impotence. J Urol 1982; 128: 45
32. Jones W J. The evaluation and treatment of psychosexual dysfunction in men. AUA Update Ser 1984; 3, Lesson 33: 1–7
33. Cookson M S, Nadig P W. Long term results with vacuum constriction device. J Urol 1993; 149: 290
34. Lue T F, Tanagho E A. Physiology of erection and pharmacological management of impotence. J Urol 1987; 139: 27
35. Sidi A A, Cameron J S, Duffy L M, Lang P H. Intracavernous drug induced erections in the management of male erectile dysfunction: experience with 100 patients. J Urol 1986; 135: 704
36. Althof S E, Turner L A, Levin S B et al. Why do so many people drop out from auto-injection therapy for impotence? J Sex Marital Ther 1989; 15: 121
37. Lewis R W, Barrett D M. Modern management of male erectile dysfunction. AUA Update Ser 1995; 14, Lesson 20: 162

Delayed urological complications of renal transplantation

10

U. Maier   S. Madersbacher   M. Marberger

Introduction

Within the past decade, urological complications following kidney transplantation have significantly decreased, yet complication rates as high as 10–30% have been reported in overviews[1] (Table 10.1). The majority of complications become clinically evident within the first month following transplantation. Consequently, the literature on late urological complications is scanty[2] (Table 10.2).

The predominant aetiology of early urological complications involves urinary fistulae and lymphocoele formation, both of which can be managed endo-urologically. The leading cause of delayed urological complications is the ureteral stenosis. Shoskes et al.[3] recently reported on urological complications of 1000 consecutive renal transplantations in 812 patients with a minimum follow-up of 12 months. In their series only 19% of all ureteral obstructions were manifested in the first 6 postoperative weeks, with an overall urological complication rate of 7.1%.

At the University of Vienna, General Hospital, the kidney transplantation programme is organized cooperatively by the Departments of Surgery, Nephrology and Urology. Kidney transplantation is performed by the transplant surgeons who usually intervene if complications become evident within the early postoperative period. Postoperative surveillance is coordinated by the Department of Nephrology. The urologist is usually involved if delayed complications are evident. The authors report herein their experience with these delayed urological complications obtained within a period of 7¼ years in a consecutive series of 1415 kidney transplantations.

Patients

All patients received a cadaver kidney transplant at the Transplant Unit of the Department of Surgery, University of Vienna, Austria. Postoperative

Author†	No. of trans-plantations	Complications(%)	Mortality(%)
Prout et al., 1967	93	9.6	22.2
Straffon et al., 1968	142	24.0	20.0
MacKinnom et al., 1968	59	33.9	45.0
Martin et al., 1969	142	16.9	29.0
MacLean et al., 1969	108	29.8	46.8
Williams et al., 1979	158	20.2	37.0
Belzer et al., 1970	220	4.0	0
Starzl et al., 1970	243	10.0	21.7
Weil et al., 1971	200	11.0	68.1
Robson and Calne, 1971	147	11.5	17.6
Fjeldborg and Kim, 1972	180	27.0	?
Presto et al., 1973	148	16.2	27.8
Malek et al., 1973	94	8.5	12.5
Malek et al., 1973	1301	13.3	32.7
O'Donoghue et al., 1973	130	12.3	13.3
Barry et al., 1974	1108	14.0	30.0
Desai et al., 1974	1164	9.1	28.3
Salvatierra et al., 1974	540	0.5	0
Marx et al., 1974	1887	12.2	?
Marx et al., 1974	87	3.5	0
Colfry et al., 1974	126	11.9	28.5
Leavy et al., 1975	221	0.9	0
Dreikorn and Röhl, 1975	2433	13.2	29.9
Rainer et al., 1976	216	14.3	14.8
Dreikorn and Röhl, 1976	133	11.2	6.6
Salvatierra et al., 1977	860	3.4	0
Salvatierra et al., 1977	250	1.6	0
Smolev et al., 1977	290	10.3	9.1
Palmer and Chatterjee, 1978	1539	5.0	13.0
MacDonald et al., 1979	88	11.0	0
Waltzer et al., 1980	500	2.8	0
Goldstein et al., 1981	4307	7.3	18.0
Goldstein et al., 1981	255	8.2	0
Mundy et al., 1981	1000	12.5	22.0
Dreikorn et al., 1982	437	6.1	7.4
Sagalowsky et al., 1983	505	3.6	5.5
Loughin et al., 1984	718	13.2	8.0
Thomalla et al., 1985	3084	6.0	?
Debruyne et al., 1988	846	9.1	3.9
Sumrani et al., 1989	1097	2.5	0.2

Table 10.1. Urological complications and mortality rates of renal transplantation*

*From ref. 1 with permission.
†For details see ref. 1.

| Author† | No. of transplantations | Complications | |
		Early	Late
Starzl	234	15/23	8/23
Weil	200	16/22	6/22
Malek	94	7/8	1/8
Barry	173	14/15	1/15
Marx	87	3/3	0/3
Holden	141	15/19	4/19
Smolev	290	22/29	7/29
Salvaterra	860	21/29	8/29
Waltzer	500	12/14	2/14
Sagalowsky	505	13/18	5/18
Total	3084	138/180 (77%)	42/180 (23%)

Table 10.2. Early and late complications of renal transplantation*

*From ref. 2 with permission.
†For details see ref. 2.

surveillance was organized in collaboration with the Department of Nephrology. If urological complications were suspected, patients were referred to the Department of Urology. Between January 1987 and March 1994, surgical intervention due to delayed urological complications was necessary in 21 (15 male and six female) patients, mean age 46.1 (range 30–66) years.

Surgery was performed after a mean of 95 days (range 28–360 days, excluding three patients, who were operated on 5, 14 and 18 years after transplantation) following transplantation. Within the same time period, a total number of 1415 kidneys were transplanted at the Transplant Unit. Hence, the actual rate of *delayed* urological complications in this series was 21/1415 (1.48%). The predominant pathology was ureteral stenosis (Table 10.3).

Complication	No.
Ureteral stenosis	11
Ureteral necrosis	8
Reflux	1
Shrinking bladder	1

Table 10.3. Aetiology of delayed urological complication after renal transplantation

Ureteral necrosis consistently revealed clinical signs comparable to those of ureteral stenosis, namely an increase of serum creatinine and a dilatation of the collecting system, without signs of extravasation.

Surgical approach

Surgical approaches are summarized in Table 10.4; the mainstay of surgical reconstruction was the ureteroneocystostomy (successful in 14/15 patients).

Surgical procedure	No.
Ureteroneocystostomy (antirefluxive)	15
Ureteroureterostomy (host ureter)	3
Ureteroureterostomy (graft ureter)	1
End-to-end anastomosis	1
Bladder augmentation (plus ureteroneocystostomy)	1

Table 10.4. Surgical approaches to delayed urological complications after renal transplantation

In one case, a second intervention was necessary, owing to a proximal restenosis of the graft ureter requiring an anastomosis of graft and host ureter. In three individuals the host ureter was used for ureteroneo-cystostomy. In one particular case, one ureter of a double kidney with an ureter duplex became necrotic and was subsequently reanastomozed after resection of the necrotic segment to the second intact duplex ureter (Figs 10.1, 10.2). A proximal ureteral stenosis was present in one patient; this was managed by an end-to-end anastomosis of the graft ureter. One patient developed a bladder contracture which ultimately caused a leak between ureter and bladder. A bladder augmentation (clamp-ileocystoplasty) combined with an ureteroneocystostomy led to an excellent postoperative result (Figs 10.3, 10.4). An interesting case involved a 56-year-old man, who developed a ureteral stenosis 18 years after transplantation, with clinical signs of progressive kidney failure; until this event, graft function had been normal. After resection of the affected segment and ureteroneocystostomy, graft function returned to normal throughout the follow-up period of 12 months (Figs 10.5, 10.6).

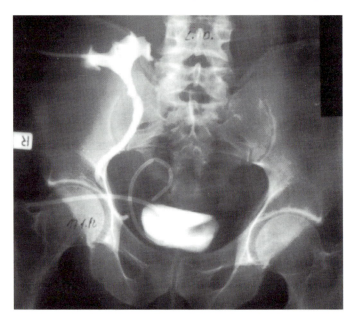

Figure 10.1. Transplant kidney with a double collecting system (preoperative). One ureter of this double collecting system became necrotic, leading to a urinoma, which was drained percutaneously.

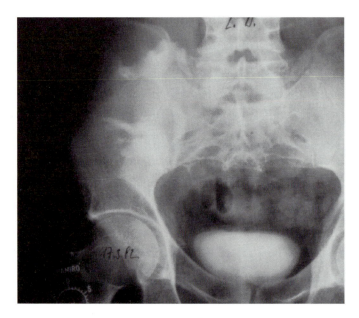

Figure 10.2. Transplant kidney with a double collecting system (postoperative). The necrotic ureteral segment has been resected and an end-to-side anastomosis of the ureters was performed.

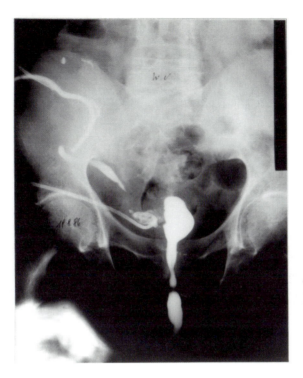

Figure 10.3. Shrinking bladder (preoperative). Owing to shrinkage of the bladder, the transplant ureter became displaced, leading to a urinoma which was drained percutaneously.

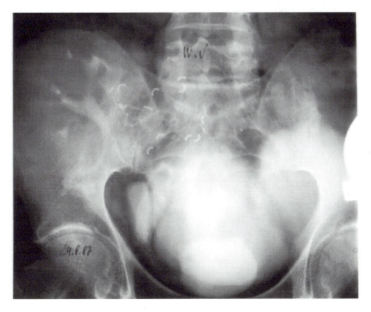

Figure 10.4. Shrinking bladder (postoperative). The bladder has been augmented and a ureteroneocystostomy achieved.

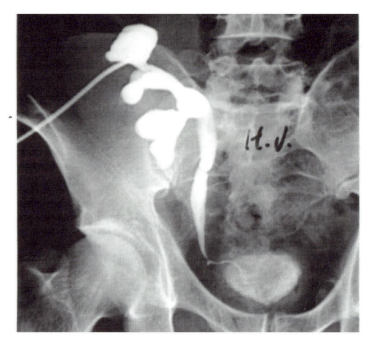

Figure 10.5. Ureteral stenosis 18 years after renal transplantation (preoperative). Note the significant prevesical stenosis, which became clinically evident 18 years after transplantation.

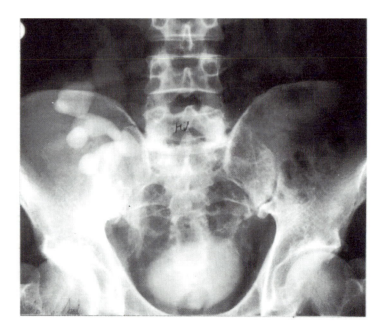

Figure 10.6. Ureteral stenosis 18 years after renal transplantation (postoperative). Postoperative result after resection of the fibrotic ureteral segment and ureteroneocystostomy.

130

Results

In the authors' series, optimal results were achieved in 19/21 patients, who were followed postoperatively for a mean of more than 2 years (Table 10.5). These patients were cured with a single surgical intervention. Graft function remained stable and serum creatinine was within normal limits. Ultrasonography consistently revealed a non-dilated urinary collecting system. The mean postoperative period of hospitalization was 12.5 days. One patient developed a recurrent severe stenosis following ureteroneocystostomy and subsequently underwent a second open surgical procedure. Reconstruction involved an anastomosis of the graft and host ureter. Graft explantation was necessary in one patient who developed severe graft rejection 4 months after ureteroneocystostomy.

Results	No.
Optimal*	19/21 (90%)
Satisfactory†	1/21
Loss of kidney graft	1/21

Table 10.5. Results (24.6 months follow-up) of surgical intervention in 21 patients with delayed urological complications after renal transplantation

*Normal serum creatinine; no dilation of collecting system; no further intervention.
†Second intervention necessary.

Conclusions

1. The rate of delayed urological complications in the authors' series (n = 1415) was 1.48% (21/1415 kidney transplantations in 7¼ years).
2. Delayed urological complications can appear as late as 18 years after transplantation.
3. Delayed urological complications after kidney transplantation require an open surgical approach, as necrotic or fibrotic ureteral segments have to be resected in order to obtain optimal results.

Discussion

Several factors have contributed to the decrease in urological complications after kidney transplantation within the past decade. Of these factors, the most important ones are improved dialysis and explantation techniques, refined immunosuppression allowing reduced cortisol doses, more sophisticated preoperative diagnostic work-up and, finally, effective endo-urological and percutaneous procedures in the cases of early urological complications. As a consequence of these improvements, the percentage of urological complications following kidney transplantation has decreased to values of 2–10% with a postoperative mortality rate close to zero.

In approximately 75% of cases the distal ureter is affected. The majority of complications occur within the first 4 postoperative weeks and, at least in the authors' hospital, are managed by the transplant surgeons. In most cases, these early complications are caused by either ureteral necrosis (which may be total, partial, short or long) or a leakage at the ureteral–bladder anastomosis. The second most frequent urological complication is a ureteral obstruction by kinking (particularly if too great a length of ureter has been left) or by lymphocoele formation. Late urological complications are predominantly caused by ureteral fibrosis or fibrosis of peri-ureteral tissue leading to ureteral compression.

The pathomechanism leading to a stenosis of the transplanted ureter several years after transplantation is not fully understood. A decreased blood supply caused by careless preparation and removal of the donor organ can almost certainly be excluded, as this would have resulted in early ureteral necrosis. Haber and Putong[4] proposed in 1965 that the ureter—being a part of the allograft—might also be subject to graft rejection, resulting in ureteral fibrosis. This theory was substantiated by Robertshaw et al.[5] and Katz et al.,[6] who demonstrated comparable alterations at the cellular and vascular level of renal parenchyma and ureter in the course of graft rejection. These rejection episodes might cause ischaemic attacks with subsequent 'immunologically' induced fibrotic reactions. Loss of ureteral elasticity might subsequently lead to stenosis but may additionally facilitate the development of a vesicorenal reflux. This presumption is supported by Dreikorn et al.,[7] who observed a significant correlation between the number of rejection episodes and the incidence of reflux development.

The principal clinical signs of a delayed urological complication following kidney transplantation are a constantly rising serum creatinine and a dilated collecting duct system, seen by ultrasonography. As a first diagnostic step, an acute or chronic graft rejection should be excluded. Subsequently, a percutaneous nephrostomy tube should be inserted. If the serum creatinine decreases, an antegrade radiological study should be performed, which usually uncovers a ureteral stenosis. Finally, the degree of obstruction is objectively assessed by a Whitaker test.

The following pathological conditions are known to lead to ureteral obstruction following kidney transplantation: oedema, extrinsic compression, ureteral stones, immunological or ischaemic fibrosis of the ureteral wall, as well as peri-ureteral fibrosis. The periurethral fibrosis is probably caused by long-term damage of the periurethral fatty tissue, induced by immunosuppression.

In the presence of ureteral obstruction and leakage, endo-urological procedures should be reserved for patients with reduced performance status, or in the acute phase when a graft rejection cannot be excluded. If this endo-urological approach is chosen, it has to be confirmed radiologically that the continuity between kidney, ureter and bladder is intact; if it is not, an open surgical approach is mandatory. In general, the success rate following endo-urological intervention ranges between 50 and 80%, and is therefore clearly less favourable than after open surgery.

It is therefore concluded that ureteral stenosis should also be considered as a potential diagnosis if creatinine levels rise, even if this occurs long after successful renal transplantation and even if ultrasonography shows only a slight hydronephrosis. If a graft rejection is excluded by biopsy or by unsuccessful cortisone-bolus therapy, a percutaneous nephrostomy tube should be placed by any means possible. Decreasing creatinine levels prove the presence of a stenosis. The definitive indication for surgical intervention is a positive Whitaker test.

The authors' retrospective data strongly suggest that endoscopic interventions (e.g. inner stenting) are not indicated in the care of delayed urological complications. The ureteral stenoses resulting from this type of fibrosis are marked and render resection of the fibrotic ureteral segment mandatory.

References

1. Dreikorn K. Problems of distal ureter in renal transplantation. Urol Int 1992; 49: 76–89
2. Thomalla J V, Lingeman J E, Leapman S B, Filo R S. The manifestation and management of late urological complications in renal transplant recipients: use of the urological armamentarium. J Urol 1985; 134: 944–948
3. Shoskes D A, Hanböry D, Granston D, Morris R J. Urological complications in 1000 consecutive renal transplant patients. J Urol 1995; 153: 18–21
4. Haber M H, Putong P B. Ureteral vascular rejection in human renal transplants. JAMA 1965; 192: 157–159
5. Robertshaw G E, Madge G E, Kauffmann H M Jr. Ureteral pathology in treated and untreated renal homografts. Surg Forum 1966; 17: 236–238
6. Katz J P, Greenstein M, Hakki A et al. Transitional epithelial lesions of the ureter in renal transplant rejection. Transplantation 1988; 45: 710–714
7. Dreikorn K, Rössler W, Horsch R et al. Incidence, causes and significance of reflux in patients in endstage renal disease and after renal transplantation. Dial Transplant 1982; 11: 126–130

Index